Your Sex Life

Dr Peter Bromwich, MRCOG, Medical Director
of Midland Fertility Services
Mark Evans, MNIMH, National Institute
of Medical Herbalists

HARRAP

London

Published 1989 by
Harrap Books Limited
19-23 Ludgate Hill, London EC4M 7PD
By arrangement with Amanuensis Books Ltd

ISBN 0 245-55067-4

This book was designed and produced by
Amanuensis Books Ltd
12 Station Road
Didcot
Oxfordshire OX11 7LL
UK

Cover design: Roger King Graphic Studios
Editorial and art director: Loraine Fergusson
Senior editor: Lynne Gregory
Editor: Laila Grieg-Gran
Illustration: David Gifford, Loraine Fergusson
Photography: Mike Tattersall
Charts: Mick Brennan, Lesley Wigmore

Prime Health Ltd, a subsidiary of Municipal General Insurance Ltd (MGI) has contributed to the cost of this publication.

PRIME
HEALTH

The information contained in this book has been obtained from professional medical sources and every care has been taken to ensure that it is consistent with current medical practice. However, it is intended only as a guide to current medical practice and not as a substitute for the advice of your medical practitioner which must, on all occasion, be taken.

Contents

Sexual anatomy

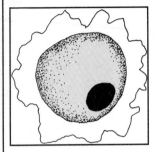

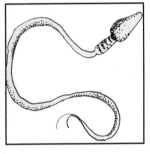

This book is about sex and the way we reproduce. It has information about the changes that occur in your body and your sex life as you mature, and age, and go through events such as pregnancy; it also has advice on keeping your sex life healthy and intact. But to describe your sex life as simply part of the system humans use to stop becoming extinct is to ignore much of what, for short, we call sex. This book discusses the organs that give you your sexual ability, the way they function, the things that can go wrong and ways, if possible, of making sure that does not happen. But the book is not just a manual about the things you can do when the moon is full. Unlike breathing, or the beating of your heart, or the way your joints work alongside each other, sex and your sex life involve strong emotions, and important cultural taboos. Your sex drive is one of the most powerful forces affecting your body; and as if this was not enough, the development of your sex life takes place at a time when there are many other changes occurring in your body, when your physical capacity for sex and love often outstrips your emotional ability to keep pace.

To start with the building blocks. Both men and women have a pair of organs (the gonads) which produce the cells that fuse together to form a new individual. These cells, called gametes, are the egg or oocyte in a woman (top), and spermatozoa in a man (below). Both sexes also have organs that protect their gametes as well as organs to make it possible for them to meet. In addition women have a uterus or womb that allows a pregnancy to grow, and breasts that are sexual organs but also nurture a baby after birth. All of these organs change dramatically at puberty (see pages 15-17).

Anatomy

In general, men are more familiar with their genital organs than women are with theirs, for two reasons. The male organs are mostly exposed, and female organs mostly concealed. Men can see themselves every time they look downwards; women need to sit on a mirror, which requires forethought, and is considered faintly disgusting by some. Even then they can't see much. Also, from childhood boys are more used to handling their genitals than girls are. Every time a boy wants to urinate he has to hold his penis in his hand to direct the flow, and then shake it and squeeze it to stop the last few drops running down his trouser leg. Girls pass urine less often than boys do, because the procedure is more complex for them. They need to squat down, rearrange their clothes, find a lavatory (it is natural and macho for boys to urinate in public, unacceptable for girls to do so). Girls are discouraged from handling their organs because they are in a 'dirty' (perhaps a better word is private) part of the body.

4

Anatomical structure gives a clue to function. The sexual anatomy of men and women is specialized, to make reproduction easier, but also to make giving and receiving pleasure possible. And pleasure is important. Humans are said to get more pleasure from sex than most other species of animal do, although how anyone knows this is a mystery. It might be because we are more intelligent, and so can justify doing things that are not necessary for our immediate survival. But it might also be that because humans are less fertile than many other species, they need to have more sex more often to reproduce than do, for example, cattle. Making sure that both partners enjoy it is one way of encouraging that. The story is not that simple; chimpanzees seem to be more fertile than humans, but also spend more of their time in all forms of sexual activity, on a fairly random basis.

There is another explanation for the fact that evolution has left us capable of enjoying sex. If sex was not fun, fewer people would enjoy it. This might seem a flippant point, but it is a serious one. Human infants are far more vulnerable than those of many animals, and sexual pleasure is one of the forces that keeps couples together, helping to provide the support of a family unit.

The sexual anatomy of men

Male sexual anatomy consists of the external organs - the scrotum and penis - and internal organs, which cannot be seen but can be felt - the testes, the prostate gland, the structures that connect them, and the accessory glands. The penis is used for urination and to deposit semen - the fluid that contains millions of spermatozoa - deep inside women.

The testis

These are sometimes called the testicles. There are two testes, and each testis is the size of a walnut. They hang outside the body in a sensitive pouch or bag called the scrotum. Most mammals have their testes outside the body because they need to be kept cooler than the rest of

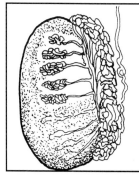

The testes feel solid, but each consists of several hundred metres of tightly packed hollow tubing. Spermatozoa (i.e. single sperm) are made by specialized cells in the lining of the tubes. As each spermatozoon is formed by the division of a basic cell it drops into the centre of the tube. From here it is carried to a specialized holding area, the epididymis, where it matures. The epididymis is another tightly folded tube, about six centimetres long, and can be felt sitting on top of the testis. It leads into the vas deferens, which carries spermatozoa to the penis.

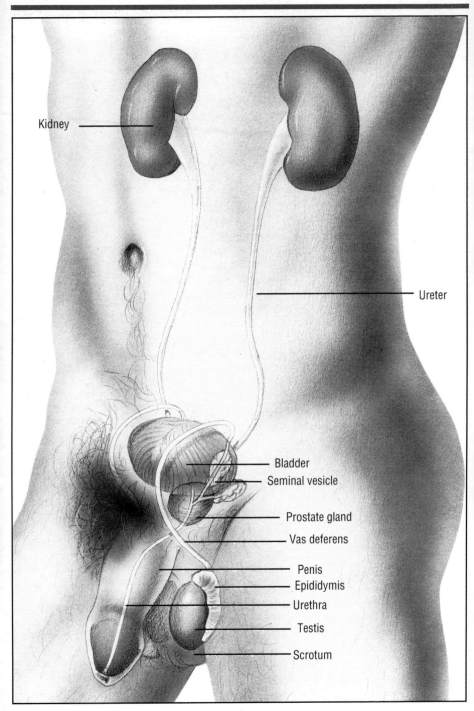

Kidney

Ureter

Bladder

Seminal vesicle

Prostate gland

Vas deferens

Penis

Epididymis

Urethra

Testis

Scrotum

the body to function properly. Most men make at least 80 million spermatozoa every day. Each spermatozoon carries half of the genetic code of the man who produced it, and when it fuses with an oocyte the new individual will have a complete set of genetic instructions, half from each parent. We are all genetically different from each other, because even brothers and sisters (except for identical twins) receive a different mix of genetic instructions from each parent.

There are two ways in which the genetic instructions of spermatozoa and oocytes differ. An oocyte is bigger than a spermatozoon, and so some additional material is carried in the oocyte. There is not much of this, and it may not have much importance after the first few hours following fertilization, but it is there.The other difference is in the sex chromosomes as described in the right-hand column.

Packed in between the tubes in the testis are other specialized cells that produce hormones. These cells are controlled by other hormones from the pituitary. The hormones from the testis are principally the androgens, the name being derived from the Greek for 'male generating'. The principal androgen is testosterone. Androgens are found in everybody, but at much higher levels in men than either women or boys. Androgens produce the changes at puberty and the sudden spurt in growth that occurs just before puberty. They also close the growing points in the bones, which ensures that your height at puberty is the tallest you ever reach, deepen the voice, enlarge the sex organs, stimulate growth of hair on the face and, unfortunately, produce teenage spots or acne.

The penis

The most obvious sexual organ in men is the penis. This is more or less a cylindrical organ that consists of the ejaculatory duct (the union of the urethra and the vasa deferentia) surrounded by three columns of specialized tissue capable of erection.

Erection

Erectile tissue resembles a dried, compressed sponge. The

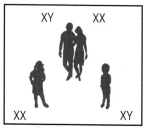

All cells in the human body contain 23 pairs of chromosomes, making 46 in all, except for the sperm and egg which have only 23 chromosomes each. When upon fertilization, the nuclei of the sperm and egg fuse, their two set of chromosomes form 46 pairs as in all other cells. The fusion of the two sets of chromosomes determines (among other things) the sex of the baby and it is the sperm that carries the deciding chromosome. All the cells in a woman's body except the eggs carry 44 non-sex chromosomes plus two X sex chromosomes. She does not have any Y chromosomes at all. Men on the other hand carry and X and a Y chromosomes on every cell in their body except the sperm, half of which carry an X, half a Y. There is no reliable way of altering the ratio of X to Y spermatozoa, although that has not stopped people searching for a method for centuries. The reading list at the end of this book has an article on this subject.

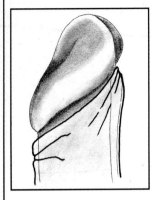

The tip of the penis (the glans) has a great many nerve endings, which makes it very sensitive to touch and pressure. It is covered by a layer of skin, the prepuce or foreskin. Circumcision (the removal of this tag of skin) was once almost routine on baby boys, but is now only practised in Britain by some religious groups, although it is still common in parts of the United States of America. In later life circumcision is sometimes done if the foreskin is diseased and, perhaps, preventing the man from passing urine, or making his erection painful or impossible.

blood vessels supplying it behave as if they have valves controlled by nerves. When these nerves are stimulated the arteries increase the amount of blood flowing into the erectile tissue. This compresses the veins which are thin-walled and so decreases the amount of blood that can flow out. The erectile tissue fills with blood, and erection begins. The stimulation that provides this can come from the brain; sexual thoughts or the sight of something or someone attractive is sufficient. There are other ways of making an erection happen. Directly stimulating the penis triggers a reflex response that is controlled through the spinal cord and produces an erection. This means that touching or massaging the penis makes it become erect, even in men who are not feeling aroused, or who have had damage to the spinal cord, and so cannot send impulses from their brain to the rest of the body. Similarly, the stimulation of nerves that a full bladder produces also leads to an erection. Erection can follow the injection of drugs that act on the walls of blood vessels directly into the penis (see page 71). This is a form of treatment that helps men unable to have an erection because of disease or damage to either the nerves or blood vessels of erectile tissue.

With erection the penis becomes swollen, firm, and starts to point upwards rather than simply hanging loosely. Incidentally, although penises vary enormously in size and shape, there is little difference between them when they are erect. Even if there was, it would not matter. The vaginal muscles will grasp firmly any size of penis. The important sensation that the vagina detects is the firmness of the erection, which depends on how well aroused the man is.

Many people feel that an erect penis must have a bone; they are sure that a simple increase in the amount of blood flowing into the penis cannot produce an erection. In fact only dogs and whales have bones in the penis, and the action of blood flowing into the human penis, and making it grow, become firm, and straight, and move, is rather similar to the way that a hosepipe filling with water swells, and becomes rigid, when the tap is opened but the outlet closed.

There are other structures that are less visible, but contribute to semen (the fluid produced by men at orgasm that helps to deliver spermatozoa to women). These include the seminal vesicles, which produce about two-thirds of the volume of semen, and the bulbo-urethral glands, the function of which is unknown, but which produce a few drops of fluid during sexual arousal.

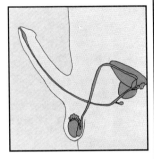

The sexual anatomy of women

Women have similar organs to men, but there are important functional and anatomical differences. Their gonads - the ovaries - produce a more complex mixture of hormones than the testes do, and instead of producing many millions of spermatozoa a day they produce one oocyte a month. Women's internal organs consist of the ovaries, the uterus or womb, the fallopian tubes that are a conduit between the two, and the vagina, which receives the penis, and so provides a channel for spermatozoa to enter the body and start their journey towards the oocyte. The external organs are the clitoris (anatomically similar to the penis, but smaller and without the urethra), and the inner and outer lips of the vagina (the labia minora and majora). The external organs are collectively known as the vulva (see page 24). Across the entrance to the vagina a thin membrane known as the hymen or maidenhead develops. This is of no anatomical importance. It is perforated to allow menstrual fluid to escape, and it usually breaks during childhood years, either following masturbation or the use of tampons. Traditionally, it was not meant to be broken until the first attempt at intercourse on the wedding night, and in some societies if the bed-sheet from that first night was not blood-stained the groom was entitled to compensation from his bride's father.

The ovary

Shortly after she has been conceived, and long before she is born, a baby girl has all the oocytes she will ever produce in her life. From then on the process is one of wastage, until at about the age of fifty the menopause (see page 39)

The ejaculatory duct
Each epididymis leads into a duct called the vas deferens. This runs just under the skin of the scrotum, and can be felt as a cord leading away from the testis. It travels upwards to the prostate, which is a small gland at the base of the bladder. Here the two vasa deferentia join with the urethra, the outlet from the bladder, to form the ejaculatory duct that runs from there along the length of the penis to the tip.

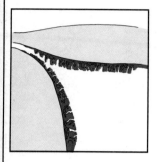

The uterus is lined by the endometrium. Every month a new lining is prepared, ready to receive a pregnancy. If there is no pregnancy the lining is shed, and a new one grows in its place. This monthly shedding of the endometrium is menstruation, also called the monthly period, or simply the period. The term 'the curse' is still sometimes used.

marks the time when all her oocytes have been used up, and the reproductive phase of her life is over. The sexual phase continues, and can even improve.

Each month a group of oocytes is chosen by the body to start to develop. The signals that control the development of them are carried by hormones (chemical messengers). Several oocytes start to develop, but usually one becomes dominant. Each oocyte develops in a fluid-filled blister (a follicle) on the surface of the ovary. The follicle is lined with hormone-secreting cells, and is discussed further on page 15. As the follicle grows the amount of hormone it produces increases almost exponentially, and this rapid surge in hormone output feeds back to the pituitary the information that all is going well, and so production of hormones to act on the ovary decreases. The ovarian hormones are also carried to the uterus (see below) where they act on the lining to make it grow.

The uterus, cervix and endometrium

The uterus or womb is a firm muscular organ that for most of a woman's life is no more than the size and shape of a small pear. During pregnancy it grows, and during labour the muscle in it contracts and squeezes out the baby and the placenta (the afterbirth).

The neck, or narrow end, of the uterus is the cervix. The cervix helps to keep a pregnancy inside the womb, but opens in labour to allow the baby out. Because it lies between the main body of the uterus and the vagina it also acts as a barrier between the internal organs and the outside world. Mucus secreted by the cervix helps to keep bacteria away from the internal organs, and when a woman is fertile, mucus helps to keep spermatozoa alive and ready for fertilization. The cervix consists of tough fibrous tissue covered by a thin layer of mucus-secreting cells with a surface that is piled into hills and valleys.

Because of the position of the cervix it is vulnerable to infections, but it is also easy for doctors to examine it for signs of disease. The cervical smear is such an examination, when a sample of the cells covering the cervix is smeared away and tested for infections or the early signs

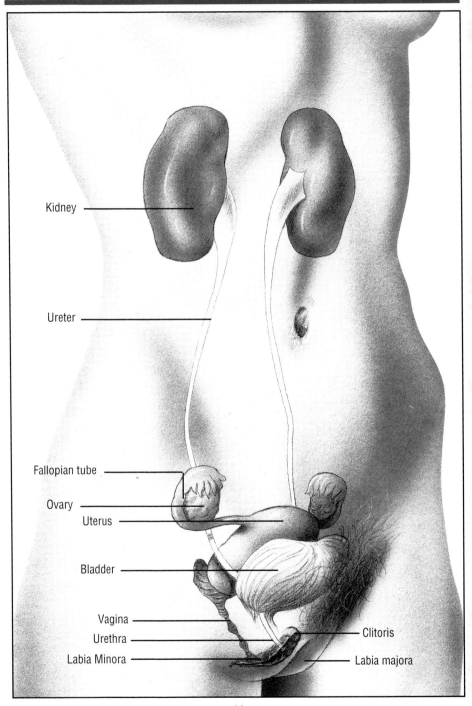

Kidney

Ureter

Fallopian tube

Ovary

Uterus

Bladder

Vagina

Urethra

Labia Minora

Clitoris

Labia majora

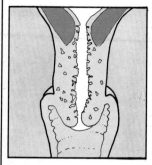

The cervix consists of tough fibrous tissue covered by a thin layer of mucus-secreting cells with a surface that is piled into hills and valleys.

of cancer. The mucus produced by the cervix is biochemically similar to that produced in the lung, and so it is hardly surprising that the same things that damage the lung also damage the cervix, since they are carried there by the bloodstream. This is one reason why cancer of the cervix is commoner amongst women who smoke cigarettes, or who live with others who smoke cigarettes, than it is among non-smokers.

The fallopian tube

The fallopian tube is shaped rather like an old-fashioned hearing trumpet. The wide end has many frond-like filaments which waft the egg from the surface of the ovary into the tube. When the muscles of the tube contract they make the tube writhe slowly, and since the inside of the tube is lined with millions of tiny hairs that beat and make a continuous current, the two movements together mean the oocyte is carried towards the uterus, but also delayed for a few days at the narrow end of the fallopian tube before entering the uterus. It is during this delay that the oocyte is fertilized, and the endometrium changes to become receptive.

The vagina

The vagina is a remarkable organ. The easiest way to illustrate it is to draw it as an open tube. It isn't really; it is more of a space that is usually closed but can stretch to receive a penis coming in, or the baby going out. It consists of a layer of muscle surrounded by a delicate lining. There are a lot of blood vessels just under the lining, which are important for intercourse (see page 23). The cells lining the vagina are continually being shed and renewed. This gives most women a regular clear non-smelly discharge that usually does not concern them. The dead cells that the body sheds have a close relationship with a specialized vaginal bacterium, the lactobacillus, an organism more usually associated with making yoghurt. This organism breaks down the cells to produce lactic acid, which kills most types of harmful bacteria, and helps to keep the vagina healthy. One unfortunate consequence of taking antibiotics, which are designed to kill bacteria, is that the lactobacilli may be killed as well, leaving the vagina susceptible to other infections.

The external organs
The external genital organs in women are not as obvious as they are in men, although since most societies regard the breasts as sexual organs, this means that, overall, women have more obvious sexual organs than men. The external genital organs consist of the mound of Venus which is the pad of fat lying under the pubic hair, the clitoris, and the inner and outer lips of the vagina which conceal the entrance to the vagina, and also have a sexual function themselves.

The breasts
There are many nerves that supply the nipple, although their main function is to help in the process of breastfeeding rather than aid sexuality. Muscle fibres under the nipple and areola help the nipple become erect which can be after a sexual stimulus, or a baby sucking, or simply something physical such as cold weather. When the nipple is stimulated the nerve impulses created act on the hypothalamus to produce the hormone oxytocin which is carried by the bloodstream back to the breast to squeeze the muscles around the milk glands and force milk out through the ducts. This means that when a baby sucks women get the 'milk-let-down' reflex, and milk dribbles from both nipples. Some get the reflexes when their baby cries to be fed.

Nipple sucking also causes the hypothalamus to release the hormone prolactin, which acts on the ovary to stop it producing oocytes (see page 34-5).

The menstrual cycle
One of the most fundamental differences between humans and most other animals is the menstrual cycle. This is the regular way in which women prepare for pregnancy, and if pregnancy does not happen, shed the old endometrium so that a new one can develop. The cycle is controlled by

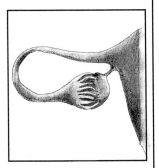

The fallopian tube runs from the body of the uterus to the ovary. The end of the tube does not completely enclose the ovary, but the frond-like fingers of it hover around the ovary to waft the released egg into the funnel and down the tube itself.

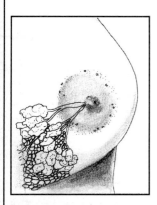

The breasts are made from a mixture of fatty tissue and glands that secrete milk. At the centre of each breast is a nipple surrounded by a flattened area called the areola. There are about 20 tiny openings into the nipple, where the milk-ducts open. Each milk-duct represents the opening from one of the 20 lobules that a breast is made of.

hormones from the hypothalamus, which act on the ovary to produce other hormones which in turn act back on the hypothalamus to make a cycle that is broken only by pregnancy, the menopause, the contraceptive pill, or some diseases.

Discussion of the menstrual cycle usually begins with menstruation. This is the time when the hormones from the ovary and the pituitary are at a low level, and the old endometrium is being shed. On average a menstrual period lasts for between three and seven days, and there is one a month. The period is a mixture of blood, mucus, and broken down cells, with a few hormones and similar things thrown in as well. Each period has a volume of 50-100 mls, and so the total volume of blood throughout a year would probably only fill a milk-bottle or two. This mixture of blood and debris is collected either on external pads, called sanitary towels, that are worn between the vulva and the pants, or on tampons, which are worn internally in the vagina. The method used is one of individual preference.

Even before a period is over the hypothalamus starts to produce the hormones that act on the pituitary to make it control the ovary and develop a new oocyte. As each oocyte grows the cells of the follicle in which it grows start to produce hormones. The principal hormone produced is oestrogen, which has many effects on the whole body, and stimulates the growth of a new endometrium. As the ovarian follicle develops it produces more and more oestrogen, which acts on the hypothalamus and pituitary to stop them producing the hormones that stimulate the follicles to grow. The rising levels of oestrogen also trigger the sudden burst of a second hormone, luteinizing hormone (LH) which has several functions. LH changes the action of the follicle cells so that they produce progesterone rather than oestrogen, and it makes the covering of the follicle burst, so that the egg can be released.

The burst follicle collapses in on itself. By this time the cells have switched to producing almost only progesterone, and this biochemical change makes the cells change colour, to bright yellow. The mass of cells, which started

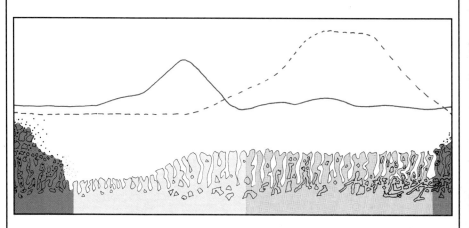

out deep in the centre of the ovary, are now on the outside, and resemble a smear of butter on the outside of the ovary. This is called the corpus luteum, which is simply Latin for yellow body.

The hormone progesterone acts on the endometrium, and makes it become thicker, and more complex, so that it begins to resemble glands. Although there are no glands in the endometrium, because the change is so characteristic, the changed endometrium is called secretory. This type of endometrium is necessary for a pregnancy.

If the oocyte is fertilized, the embryo that forms will travel down the fallopian tube, reaching the uterus about five days after the oocyte left the ovary. The embryo immediately sends chemical signals to the ovary, so that the cells of the corpus luteum continue to produce progesterone, and keep the endometrium steady. If this does not happen, the corpus luteum begins to die, stops producing progesterone, the endometrium loses the hormone signals that keep it healthy, and so it dies, and is shed by the body as menstruation. A new cycle has begun.

Puberty

Puberty is the process that children go through as they become adults. It is not something that happens overnight,

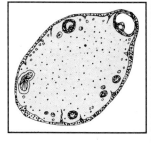

The developing follicle , which can be seen top right of the ovary, releases increasing quantities of oestrogen. This in turn stimulates the endometrium to thicken. Ovulation occurs on one day of the cycle, leaving the corpus luteum (seen in the lower right portion of the ovary) which releases progesterone. Without the influence of high levels of oestrogen the endometrium begins to break up and as the level of progesterone falls, menstruation begins again.

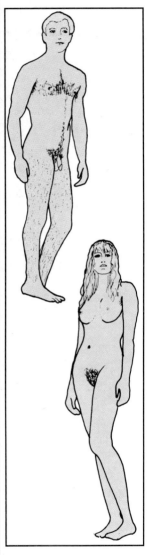

Male and female secondary sexual characteristics develop during puberty.

but is a slow progression that lasts for several years. In many societies it is marked by religious or tribal rituals. In some societies it is only at puberty that children become people; before that they are only potential people, outside the protection of society. This is still true to a limited extent in Britain; although children have full legal protection in most matters, there is no legal obligation for the authorities to provide housing for young homeless people, whereas they are required to do so for adults.

There are some features of puberty that are common to both sexes, such as the sudden spurt in growth that happens just before puberty. In both boys and girls there is a change in body shape as well as size as they assume adult proportions. Hair grows under the armpits and over the pubis, and although acne is upsetting it occurs because of the change from the more delicate skin of children to the tougher skin of an adult.

In both sexes the onset of puberty is characterized by changes in the pattern of hormones secreted by the pituitary, and certain kinds of brain damage in children can prevent puberty from taking place. Interestingly enough, light also plays a part: children blind from birth go through puberty on a different time-scale to those who are sighted, or who lost their sight comparatively late.

Puberty in boys

Pubertal changes in boys are caused by the development of the testes, which grow, and produce more of the male hormones, called androgens. Androgens have many functions. They make hair grow, particularly on the face, and under the armpits, and on the pubis, but to a lesser extent on the legs and the rest of the body. They deepen the voice. They are anabolic, in other words, they increase the amount of muscle mass, and they appear to increase growth. The banned steroids that some athletes take are of a similar type,and have a similar effect, although because these are synthetic they can be made many times more powerful. They are also designed to increase only muscle mass, but since they also depress the body's own hormone production, they cause the athlete's testes to shrivel,

16

among other side-effects.

All of these hormone effects come from the testis. Many years ago cathedral choirs consisted of castrati. These were singers who as boys had had their testes removed, to prevent them from going through puberty. This meant that their voices did not deepen, and so they kept the singing voice of a young boy forever.

The fact that the testis was the source of these effects was recognized by the Romans. Only men were allowed to testify in court and before the Senate, and speakers were examined to make sure that not only did they have testes, but that these were of a sufficient size to ensure that the owner was in fact a man, and not a boy. Two testes testified to the qualifications of the speaker; hence the similarity between testicle, testament and testify. Incidentally, it was not only the ancient Romans who insisted that only men with testes had authority. Legend has it that the furore over Pope Joan meant that all future candidates for the papacy were inspected before selection. They would sit on a marble throne with a hole in the base, and be examined by a courtier, who would feel for testes; if he found none they could not be elected.

A girl's first period is usually between her eleventh and fourteenth birthday, although some girls start having regular menstrual periods when they are only eight, and others not until they are sixteen. The age of the girl is not the most important factor: her onset of puberty is related to her size, weight, and the amount of fat she has in her body. Young girls who starve themselves, or have many hours a day of rigorous exercise, delay the onset of puberty.

Puberty in girls

Puberty in girls is more complex. As in boys, there are some obvious changes, such as the breasts developing, and more subtle ones. In boys the voice 'breaks' and becomes deeper and gruffer, but the change in girls is less obvious, although still there. The most important developments are concealed, but the maturing of the external genitals is accompanied by fundamental changes in the internal organs.

From about the age of eight the pituitary gland starts producing pulses of hormone that act on the ovary to start oocytes developing. As the ovaries become able to release oocytes the final stages of puberty begin. A girl's first menstrual period is usually preceded by a clean, whitish vaginal discharge for a few months. This discharge is made up of dead cells thrown out by the growing uterus, cervix, and vagina.

Sexual physiology

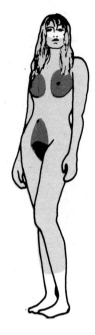

Female erogenous zones

So, once the necessary organs have developed, what next? Sexual activity is possible at almost any age, from baby-hood upwards, but fertility occurs only after puberty and, in women, before the menopause. Sexual physiology is a fairly boring term for the way that men and women become aroused, and find sexual relief. This need not necessarily be with each other; the body's responses are the same for a solitary person masturbating, as they are for two people of the same or opposite sex making love, or having sex, or enjoying intercourse, or whatever term you wish to use.

Masturbation and oral sex

From a scientific viewpoint there is little difference be-tween masturbation and intercourse. At a physiological level both are a means of achieving orgasm, and an orgasm is an explosive release of sexual tension. Masturbation usually implies self-stimulation, although for many couples mutual masturbation (masturbation of each other) is part of lovemaking. Intercourse is the use of the genitals of one person to penetrate those of another.

Masturbation

Masturbation is common. Most surveys suggest that almost everybody masturbates at some stage of their lives, and it could be argued that never to masturbate is almost as unusual as to rely entirely on masurbation for sexual enjoyment. Masturbation is the manipulation of the geni-tals, usually using your hands, but often with a variety of implements to help. It is a common practice, found in all age groups from babies to the elderly, although to read some of the medical literature of last century or early this century you would never believe it was a normal and healthy activity.

Oral sex

The mouth and lips are important for sexual pleasure. For most couples kissing is a prelude to lovemaking, and oral sex is simply transferring that behaviour to the genitals. Cunnilingus is oral sex involving the genitals of a woman, and fellatio those of a man. The French term soixante-neuf (69) is commonly used to describe the situation when a couple are simultaneously stimulating each other orally. (It is called 69 not because there are only 68 other ways for giving each other pleasure, but because two people lying together in this position are said to resemble the number 69). There is nothing wrong with oral sex, but it can be a bit frightening when you first try it. At least it can't make you pregnant! In theory it could get you into trouble: like many aspects of life the law has not caught up with the behaviour of most of the population, and there are some parts of the world where oral sex is considered illegal. The laws are not enforced.

Foreplay

Foreplay is simply a term for the stimulation of someone before, or instead of, intercourse, and part of the enjoyment of sex comes in ways of stimulating and arousing your partner.

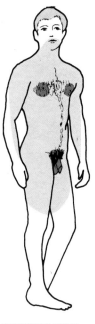

Male erogenous zones

Sexual intercourse, sex, coitus, making love

Intercourse is another word for communication, which few people seem to realize. Sexual intercourse is just one of the many ways two people communicate love and enjoyment with each other. The reactions and responses of those people are the same if they are of the same or different sexes, and there is little difference between the physiological responses shown by two strangers or two long-term lovers. Most people achieve sexual gratification with a mixture of intercourse and masturbation, sometimes at the same time.

The physiology of sexual intercourse is remarkably similar for men and women, with a few important differences. Scientists divide intercourse into four stages: arousal, excitement, plateau, and orgasm, which are followed by resolution. The terms are simple enough: the

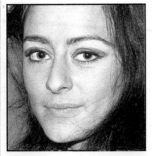

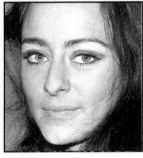

The pupils of your eyes dilate when you are interested in something or someone. Compare the two photographs. Which of the twins is the more interesting, or the more attractive? Both photographs are of the same woman, and are actually printed using the same negative. But the one above has been photographically retouched to make the pupils appear larger. Most people feel that this sign, which simply means that you find what you are looking at interesting, makes you appear more attractive, friendlier, and altogether a nicer person.

behaviour of the body is more complex.

The early stages are the same in both sexes. Arousal can follow sexual thoughts, or the appreciation of someone attractive. Some men and women, especially the young, are easily aroused. The sensation that causes the arousal might be the sight or sound of someone, or simply something that triggers a memory, such as the smell of perfume or after-shave lotion. Or simply the smell of his or her body. Natural body smells are individual, and important sources of arousal for many people. Arousal can follow something purely physical, such as manipulation of the genitals or something entirely intellectual. In both men and women similar things happen, the eyes widen which has a number of effects as can be seen from the photographs in the left-hand column.

The drug atropine also dilates the pupil, and so is used by eye specialists. The deadly nightshade plant contains atropine-like substances, and so extracts of it were once used by society ladies to make them more attractive to men (hence the botanical name of the plant, belladonna). Don't try this yourself; apart from the fact that it is dangerous and can lead to death or blindness, there are other much better ways of making yourself attractive.

Obviously nobody measures the size of the pupils of the person they are talking to. All of these points are tiny ones, and most are recognized by our subconscious rather than being actively looked for, although you can train yourself to observe them. They are part of what is called 'body-language', and in matters of love and sexual behaviour they are usually much more important than the words we use.

Along with these signs are other more medical ones that both men and women show. The pulse rate often increases, and sometimes becomes irregular. The rate at which you breathe increases.

Sexual physiology of men

In men the increased blood-flow to the penis produces an erection. Erection occurs rapidly during the arousal phase and leads to the excitement phase. For many men the arousal phase is short. Erection makes a penis grow larger and become firmer, although it is quite common for the size and degree of firmness to fluctuate.

The size of the flaccid (unerect) penis varies between men, but interestingly enough the size of the erect penis is remarkably similar between different men. In other words, penises that are smaller than average when non-erect grow proportionally more when they are becoming erect. The changes in the body during excitement are not limited to the penis. The skin of the scrotum becomes thicker, and the testes are lifted up towards the body. Some men get erections of their nipples, and many men find that their nipples become much more sensitive to stimulation at this time.

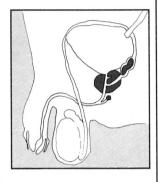

Ejaculate is made up of fluid from the prostate gland, the seminal vesicles and the bulbo-urethral glands, all of which lie below the bladder. This fluid contains the spermatozoa.

The sexual tension of the excitement phase leads into the plateau phase. There is some increase in size of the penis during this phase, particularly around the glans, which often changes colour as it becomes engorged with blood, and takes on a reddish/bluish/purplish hue. This phase can be short for many men, and there is a great deal of variation in the length of this phase between one man and another, or for the same man on different occasions.

There are other changes that occur. A rash, looking rather like that of measles, appears on the face and chest. Small muscles in the scrotum lift the testes up still higher and closer to the body, and they also begin to swell.

The plateau phase leads into a stage of 'ejaculatory inevitability'. This is one of those sensations that is difficult to describe, but is recognized by any man who has had it. Like so many things in life, if you have to have the sensation explained to you, you would not recognize it anyway. It occurs when semen moves from the seminal vesicles and prostate, into the ejaculatory duct prior to ejaculation. It is a point of no return, because once a man feels this sensation then ejaculation and orgasm are inevitable.

In both men and women the orgasm (also called the climax, or simply 'coming') is considered important. Learned tomes were once written emphasizing that the

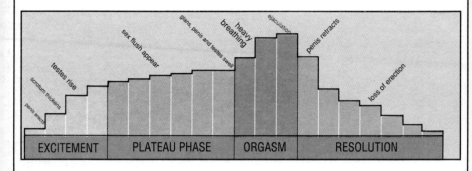

Stages of sexual excitement in men.

ideal relationship was one where both partners climaxed simultaneously. Few people believe this now.

The orgasm in men coincides with ejaculation. It is a series of rhythmic contractions of the prostate gland, the muscles of the pelvis, and the shaft of the penis. These contractions occur at the same frequency in men and women, although women usually have more. The muscles around the base of the bladder are closed shut, and so the semen is forced forward, and out of the tip of the penis, rather than into the bladder. The different components of the ejaculate - the spermatozoa, the fluid from the prostate and seminal vesicles, and the secretion from the bulbo-urethral glands - are only mixed together in the ejaculatory duct, and so there are marked differences in chemical composition between the fluid that is ejaculated at the beginning of orgasm, and the fluid at the end, even though the whole process is over in a matter of seconds. The average ejaculate contains from 20 to 300 million sperma-tozoa, and is rarely enough to fill a teaspoon.

After orgasm comes resolution, where one of the major differences between men and women becomes apparent. After orgasm, men have a refractory phase, during which further sexual stimulation is not possible, and may even be painful. For young men, this phase may last for only a few minutes, but for older men it may last several hours. After orgasm the erection fades away in two phases. Initially it is lost rapidly, and this is followed by a second slower phase of shrinking. This change in size of

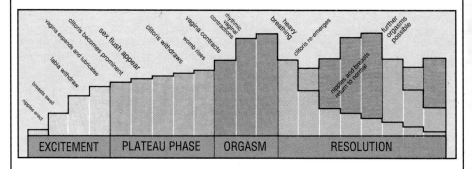

EXCITEMENT | PLATEAU PHASE | ORGASM | RESOLUTION

Stages of sexual excitement in women.

the penis is important, because after ejaculation as the penis shrinks back to its normal size there may be leakage of semen from around the edge of a condom.

Sexual physiology of women

There are many remarkable similarities between the physiology of sexual intercourse in men and women. The same stages - arousal, excitement, plateau, orgasm, and resolution occur, and the underlying physiological mechanisms are similar.

Arousal follows the same process in women as in men, although the sorts of stimuli that women find erotic are not usually the same as those that arouse men. In addition, sexual interest in women is more dependent on environmental factors than it is in men. A woman's capacity for arousal changes during her menstrual cycle, as well as depending on her general hormonal status, her age and the type of relationship she is in. The major hormonal changes associated with pregnancy and childbirth affect sexual desire and sexual behaviour in women.

During the excitement phase in women there is an increase in blood flow to the pelvis, but, as in men, signs of excitement are visible in many other parts of the body. Vaginal lubrication occurs less than 30 seconds after sexual stimulation starts. Vaginal lubrication comes from a process remarkably similar to that which causes erection in men. More blood flows to the vagina, whilst less flows away, and the congestion leads to an ooze of fluid from the

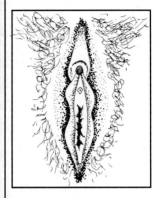

The vulva is the external female organs which include the labia majora on the outside, the labia minora on the inner edge, and the clitoris (highlighted). The vaginal opening can be seen at the base of the illustration, the urethral opening between the vagina and the clitoris.

whole vaginal surface. This process is misunderstood by many. There are several small glands at the entrance to the vagina which were once thought to be important for lubrication. They are not. Lubrication occurs rapidly, and internally, so if the woman or her partner does not bring any of the fluid to the outside she may seem unaroused.

Whilst this is happening the glans of the clitoris (the analogue in woman of the glans of the penis in men) swells, and the shaft of the clitoris grows and becomes erect. The vagina begins to balloon as the upper two-thirds expands and distends. The uterus is also lifted upwards, and many women find their nipples become erect.

The excitement phase leads to the plateau phase. Unlike men, this phase naturally has peaks and troughs, and so some women find their level of sexual tension beginning to fall after a rise, which may make them feel as if they are 'going off the boil'. This is a natural phenomenon, but some women get worried by it, sometimes so worried that they feel inhibited and try to avoid further arousal, or even situations when this might happen. Once you think you are failing in something as important as sex, a common response is never to try again.

As in men, women get a rash, which again looks rather like that of measles, over their face and chest, and there is an increase in blood flow to the pelvis. Their breasts become larger, and the areolae (the darkish area around the nipple) become engorged with blood, which can give the areola a red or bluish tinge.

The most prominent changes in women follow the increase in blood flow to the pelvis. The lower one-third of the vagina swells, making the entrance to the vagina narrower increasing the pressure on the penis. The upper two-thirds of the vagina continues to balloon outward. The clitoral head and shaft withdraws into the hood of the clitoris. The clitoris often becomes extremely sensitive at this time and most women say that direct pressure on it is painful. The labia minora (the inner lips to the vagina) show a dramatic change in colour, and become a deep red colour that has been likened to that of ruby port wine.

Orgasm in women follows a similar pattern to that

of men. There are a series of contractions of the lower one-third of the vagina which gradually fade away, and sometimes there are other involuntary spasms of muscles elsewhere in the body. In some women there is a small leakage of fluid from the urethra; this may be urine or it might be fluid from one of the glands around the urethra. Nobody knows the functions of these glands, or why this secretion of fluid at orgasm happens.

As in men, orgasm in women is followed by resolution, and a feeling of well-being. Again, there are differences between the sexes. Many men feel tired after orgasm, and want to either rest or sleep. Women have the same feeling of relaxation and well-being after orgasm but they want to share this with their partner. Unfortunately, they often want to talk and be close whilst their partner may not feel like doing anything but sleeping.

Psychiatrists once felt that there were differences between the vaginal orgasm and the clitoral orgasm: an orgasm achieved in women by masturbation was said to be immature, and the only fulfilling orgasm was one that followed direct penetration of the vagina by the penis. Unhappily for theorists, the orgasm is the same however it is achieved, and all develop from the clitoris anyway. The differences reported relate more to the feelings of the couple for each other, and their ability to communicate in ways other than intercourse.

Fertility

The beginning of this section mentioned reproduction. Sex is not only about reproduction, it is also about trying not to become pregnant or make someone pregnant. The remainder of this section will be about fertility, and infertility, contraception, and pregnancy, with a short discussion on the menopause.

Infertility

It may seem surprising, but humans are not a terribly efficient race at breeding. Most times that most couples have intercourse without using contraception a baby does

In men the plateau phase usually leads into orgasm, and the same can happen in women, after a similar phase of ejaculatory inevitability. But there are three possible variants.

• The plateau phase can be prolonged. There can be several peaks of sexual excitement, each followed by a relative trough. Prolonged plateau phase occurs more often in women than in men.

• For some women, and more so for women than for men, the plateau phase can lead directly into resolution, so that there is sexual excitement without orgasm following it.

• The plateau phase can lead into orgasm, and before resolution there is another plateau immediately followed by several more orgasms. This is perhaps the most important difference between the sexes; men are usually capable of only one orgasm before they enter a refractory phase during which they are incapable of further stimulation, and may even find attempts at arousal uncomfortable, whilst many women are capable of, and enjoy, multiple orgasms.

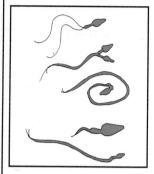

In any normal ejaculate a certain percentage of the sperm will have abnormalities like those shown above. These prevent them swimming up to the ovum. If a man's ejaculate contains more than 25% abnormal sperm, or if the number of sperm is lower than 100 million, a man is classed as subfertile.

not result. At best, there is only a 25% or so chance of a baby, even if a perfectly fertile couple have intercourse on the most fertile day of a cycle. (The chances of a pregnancy are slightly higher, because many pregnancies fail before they produce a baby.) This means that many couples who stop using contraception to have a baby are disappointed after the first month, but usually achieve their ambition after a relatively short time. But there are some who do not.

Male fertility problems

Fertility problems on the male side of a relationship can be caused by him producing no spermatozoa, or too few spermatozoa, or unhealthy spermatozoa, or being unable to ejaculate those spermatozoa into his partner. There is usually little that can be done if infertility is caused by the first three problems, either to prevent these problems from happening or to treat them once they have developed. Infections of the genital tract are discussed in the next section of this book, but one complication they can have is to cause scarring and blockage of the ejaculatory system, usually either at the epididymis or shortly after it becomes the vas deferens. Inability to ejaculate, or ejaculation before vaginal penetration (premature ejaculation), is discussed on page 65.

One common treatment for male fertility problems is artificial insemination with donor semen (AID or DI). In this process semen from an anonymous donor is put into the cervical mucus of a woman trying to conceive. The procedure is simple, but can lead to problems. With care, most of the obvious ones, such as infection, can be prevented but the difficulties that remain are important. These include sexual difficulties between the couple, because fertility and the ability to make someone pregnant are closely linked by many people in most societies with potency and the ability to have intercourse; if self-esteem in either partner falls, sexual difficulties often follow. Similarly, some men find it difficult to make love with their partner if they feel semen from another man is still inside her. All of these problems can be distressing, but with care, and understanding, and discussion, they can be lessened. This process is called counselling, and couples usually receive it before they start this fertility treatment. It is discussed in greater detail in section three.

Female fertility problems

Female fertility problems are broadly similar to, and as common as, male fertility problems. Women can be unable to produce oocytes (eggs), or they produce them too infrequently, or of too poor a quality. They may have a blockage in the fallopian tube or have cervical mucus that does not allow spermatozoa to survive long enough to meet an oocyte. Additionally, some women are unable to tolerate vaginal intercourse.

The commonest cause of not ovulating is being underweight, and once this problem has been corrected most women who have stopped ovulating return to normal. If they do not, good treatment is now possible. Treatment of ovulation difficulties has changed dramatically over the past 20 years. There are now effective fertility drugs that directly or indirectly stimulate the ovary to produce oocytes, although if these drugs are not given carefully they can make the ovary over-respond, and produce several oocytes at once, with the risk of a multiple birth.

There is not much (yet) that can be done to help the problem of absent or poor quality cervical mucus, apart from bypassing the cervix through treatment such as in vitro fertilization (the test-tube baby technique). Similarly, blocked fallopian tubes (a consequence of the infections discussed on page 47) can be helped surgically or bypassed using the same technique. Vaginismus (spasm of the pelvic muscles so severe as to prevent entry of the penis) can be helped (see page 63).

Any problem with infertility can lead to sexual unhappiness. If you believe that the only reason for having intercourse no longer exists or will no longer produce the desired result, then part of the basis for your relationship is lost. Again, care and counselling are an integral part of most fertility treatments.

A couple are said to be infertile if they have had no pregnancy after a year or so of regular intercourse without contraception. Infertility can follow problems with the man, problems with the woman, problems with both, or be inexplicable.

Contraception

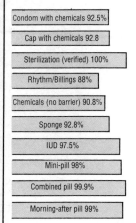

Condom with chemicals 92.5%

Cap with chemicals 92.8

Sterilization (verified) 100%

Rhythm/Billings 88%

Chemicals (no barrier) 90.8%

Sponge 92.8%

IUD 97.5%

Mini-pill 98%

Combined pill 99.9%

Morning-after pill 99%

Throughout history most sexual activity has been for recreation rather than procreation. The difference between now and prehistory is that rather than relying on luck, or primitive and unreliable methods, men and women have a range of techniques that prevent pregnancy, and in nearly every country in the world if those contraceptive methods fail there is access to simple, safe and easy abortion, although for most people this is an unpleasant option.

Using contraception is important for sexual enjoyment, and your choice of contraceptive method is a personal one. There are detailed books that will help you, and family planning clinics and your family doctor are there to guide you, but the final choice of method to use is yours. Contraception is one area of life where the only good decisions are ones that you make yourself, because only you know what your needs are, and what you feel really happy with using. Lots of science fiction novels include suggestions for mass compulsory contraception as an answer to the world's population pressures; none of these are ever likely to be successful. There was even one light-hearted suggestion that the oral contraceptive pill should be baked into every loaf of bread; as the author suggested, 'Let's take the mother out of Mother's Pride'. Your choice of contraception is personal; the guide that follows is short and simply gives you an idea of the range of choices possible.

Contraceptive methods

There is no such thing as the perfect contraceptive method, or even the best method for any one couple. You will need to use the method that suits you at the time you make your choice. When you are young, and becoming sexually active for the first time, you will probably want a method that is unlikely to fail, and which causes the absolute minimum interference with your sex life. When you are older, you might want a method that will make sure you never again become pregnant, or something that will simply delay your next pregnancy by a year or so.

The pill

The pill is perhaps the most famous contraceptive of all. It was the first successful birth control method that did not need to be fitted, or worn, or used at the time of intercourse. It consists of two hormones, an oestrogen and a drug that mimics progesterone, and both forms of hormone are effective when swallowed. There is also a progesterone only pill which can be used by women past their most fertile years (i.e. after the age of thirty-five) or by breastfeeding mothers.

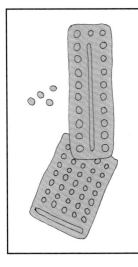

Taking the pill prevents the development of some cancers, such as cancer of the ovary and cancer of the body of the uterus, but neither of these cancers is as common as the two most important cancers of women, cancer of the lung and cancer of the breast (although no one has ever suggested a link between cancer of the lung and contraception.) There is uncertainty about the link between the pill and cancer of the cervix and cancer of the breast. There is no evidence that the modern low-dose pill causes either of these cancers, but it probably does not prevent them either. This is because cancer of the cervix might be caused by an infection carried by men, and catching this infection is prevented by using barrier contraceptives, and women who use the pill do not usually use barriers as well.

When the pill is taken regularly there is less than a two per cent chance of unwanted pregnancy in any one year of using it. It does not interfere with intercourse, which is a strength for many people because they do not want anything to ruin the spontaneity and enjoyment of sex. It is also a weakness, because contraceptives that act as a barrier to spermatozoa also prevent things other than pregnancy, such as infection. In some ways the pill acts as a barrier, because it affects cervical mucus, but it is not as effective a barrier as one made of rubber.

Cancer of the breast is commoner in women who have delayed the birth of their first child, and the pill is one important way of stopping women from becoming pregnant too early. Unfortunately, even the most modern research on the links between the pill and breast cancer are based on surveys that studied old-fashioned high-dose pills taken a long time ago. They may not be relevant to the situation of today.

The pill thickens the mucus produced by the cervix. This is an important additional benefit that helps to prevent pregnancy, and this thickened cervical mucus makes it more difficult for bacteria to pass through and reach the inner pelvic organs. Some of these infections are carried 'piggy-back' style by spermatozoa, and since the mucus of women taking the pill is temporarily hostile to spermatozoa these can no longer enter the body easily and spread the infection they are carrying.

Taking the pill does have some potentially serious complications, although these are much rarer with modern pills than they were seven to ten years ago.Oestrogen makes the blood more likely to clot in the blood vessels, and although this is uncommon in young people, it is more likely to happen in women who smoke cigarettes, or take the pill, and especially those who do both.

The pill can change moods, sometimes for the better when it prevents the symptoms of the premenstrual syndrome that so upset many women, but it may lead to an unpleasant depression. Sometimes, but not always, pill depression is lifted by taking tablets of pyridoxine (vitamin B_6). This is effective, and freely available from chemists and health-food shops. Vitamin B_6 helps many other types of hormone-associated depression. Some women get a temporary rise in blood pressure from taking the pill, and again it seems to be the oestrogen that causes this.

The intrauterine device (the IUD)

The IUD is not suitable for those women whose uterus has not yet been stretched by a pregnancy, especially those who are still young, and it does not prevent infection of the inner pelvic organs in the way that either the pill or barriers do. In fact if a woman catches a pelvic infection whilst she is using an IUD the device usually makes the consequence of the infection more severe, because the IUD acts as a septic focus for the infection. Pelvic infection (salpingitis) has severe long-term complications (see page 50).

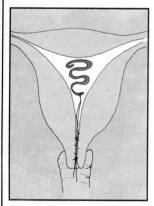

The intrauterine device is also called the coil. It is a small device made of plastic and copper, and is placed by a doctor directly into the cavity of the uterus through vagina and cervix. It sits there for several years at a time preventing pregnancy by stopping the embryo from embedding itself in the uterus.

Women who use the IUD have a between two and seven per cent chance of pregnancy every year. Some of these pregnancies are in the fallopian tubes rather than the uterus, and this is probably the most serious potential complication of using the IUD. Despite all this gloominess, the IUD is still a good method of contraception for many women. It does not need to be remembered, because once fitted it is always there. Most IUDs last for several years before they need changing.

Barrier contraceptives used by women

Recipes for barriers used by men and women to prevent pregnancy go back to the dawn of time. Thankfully, women no longer need to chant prayers whilst smearing crocodile dung with honey to use as a vaginal contraceptive, or cut a lemon in half to fit into the vagina before intercourse.

Barriers used by women consist of cream, jellies, and pessaries all of which kill spermatozoa, rubber caps which cover the cervix, and are usually used along with spermicidal creams, and a few experimental methods.

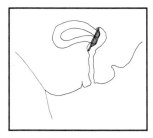

The diaphragm fits into the vagina covering part of the front wall as well as the cervix.

There are three main types of rubber barrier. The commonest is the diaphragm, or Dutch cap. This is a dome shaped, circular sheet of rubber stretched between a steel rim. It fits into the vagina, covering part of the front wall as well as the cervix. It needs to be used along with a spermicidal cream. It protects the cervix against contact with semen, and the spermicides kill bacteria as well as spermatozoa, and so prevent infection as well as pregnancy. It needs to be fitted every time you have intercourse, which some women find restrictive, but others liberating; they can choose when and with whom to use it. And they need to handle and understand their own body for the cap to be effective. It is as good a contraceptive in terms of avoiding pregnancy as the IUD, but because it needs extra care, and motivation, women who use it are slightly more likely to find themselves pregnant than those who rely on the IUD.

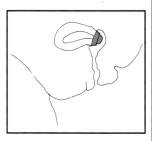

The cervical cap fits over the cervix itself and is held in place by suction.

The cervical cap is a device both old and new. For many decades it was one of the mainstays of contraceptive clinics, but with the advent of the pill it became less widely used, and in fact, almost forgotten. It is now being more widely used, but in the lean years for barrier contraception following the development of the pill the skills needed to fit it disappeared and most of the factories that made the cervical cap closed. It consists of a rubber cap resembling a large thimble containing spermicidal cream that is held against the cervix by suction. It has many of the advantages of the diaphragm, but since it is smaller the women

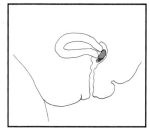

The vaginal sponge sits at the top of the vagina and covers the cervix. It is impregnated with spermicide.

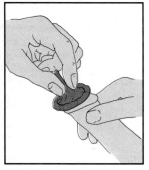

A condom should be placed on the penis before any penetration. Squeeze the air out of the end of the condom before rolling it down the full length of the penis.

who use it consider it less obtrusive. It may be a better contraceptive than the standard diaphragm, but because it is not widely used the hard evidence is lacking.

Barrier contraceptives used by men

There is only one effective barrier used by men: the condom or sheath. This has been used for millennia, but only really became widely used as a contraceptive this century. The condoms used by men several hundred years ago were thick, needed to be wet and softened before being used, and were not as efficient as the modern thin rubber condom. They were made of linen or pouches of intestine of animals, and were designed to be reused many times over. When the rubber industry developed in the second half of the last century it became possible to develop thin, strong, stretchy, rubber condoms, that were cheap enough to be disposable.

Most modern condoms are lubricated with spermicidal oil which has several functions. It makes the condom more effective as a contraceptive; any stray spermatozoa are killed by the spermicide. It also helps prevent the condom from breaking should it be used when there is some resistance to vaginal penetration, such as might happen if the woman is not fully aroused and has not produced sufficient lubrication. The lubricating oil also makes the condom a little easier to put on.

The condom, if carefully used, is a more effective contraceptive than either the cap or the IUD. But that phrase gives the clue to the biggest practical problem in using the condom. 'If carefully used'. The condom needs to be put on when a man's erection is firm enough for the rubber to be able to grip the penis, but before there has been any contact between the vagina and the penis. The condom needs to be removed as soon as ejaculation has happened, because after orgasm the penis shrinks back to its normal size, which means that the condom is no longer tight fitting, and semen can leak from the edges.

There are other advantages to condoms. They prevent contact between spermatozoa, or semen, and the cervix. Some spermatozoa carry bacteria on their outer skin, and bacteria or viruses sometimes live in semen (the fluid that spermatozoa swim in). Semen may have other substances that irritate the cervix and lead to the sort of inflammation that either needs treatment or makes the cervical smear abnormal.

Condoms don't only protect women. If a woman has a genital infection then using a condom will protect her partner. Many couples use the pill for contraception, because it is so reliable, but also use the condom, to reduce their chances of getting infections from each other.

Men who use the condom whinge about one thing. They say it interferes with sensation. They say that using the condom is like swimming with wellington boots on, or wearing a rain-coat in the shower. It is a ridiculous analogy; no condom is as thick as that! But it is a popular belief, and one that is difficult to argue against. If you believe that wearing a condom affects the sensitivity of your penis, then no amount of discussion or argument will alter your opinion.

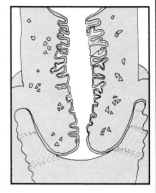

Cells within the crypts that line the cervix secrete different types of mucus at different phases of the cycle (see overleaf). Observation and careful teaching can help a woman learn her fertility cycle and plan intercourse around the days when conception is very unlikely.

Natural methods of contraception

Not every man or woman wants to avoid pregnancy using drugs or chemicals or barriers. There are lots of possible reasons for this, and lots of ways of going about it. Some simply avoid any form of risky behaviour such as vaginal intercourse at the most fertile time of the menstrual cycle, whilst others have no sexual activity at all then. Others prevent pregnancy by relying on the natural anti-fertility effect of breastfeeding. Although this depends on having had a baby quite recently!

There are three main methods of natural family planning. The first is to make sure that ejaculation does not happen in the vagina. The oldest such method is perhaps withdrawal, sometimes dignified with the name coitus interruptus. As the name implies, this is vaginal inter-course where the man pulls his penis out of the vagina as soon as he feels he is about to ejaculate.

The method is fraught with difficulties. Not all men are aware of the point of ejaculatory inevitability. When they do feel it, it is actually a sign that ejaculation has

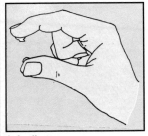

Infertile-type mucus

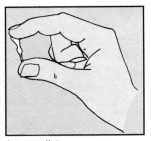

Intermediate mucus

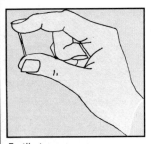

Fertile-type mucus

already begun, and so they may not have enough time to withdraw before the first spermatozoa are released. Even if a man does manage to withdraw in time, because some spermatozoa trickle into the ejaculatory system in the minutes before orgasm, there may be a risk of pregnancy from those spermatozoa that were deposited in the vagina well before ejaculation. Some textbooks also say that couples who practise withdrawal become frustrated and angry: this does not really sound likely, because if they did it would have been noticed before in clinics, and no one seems to complain of this problem in family planning clinics.

There are other similar methods. In some cultures anal intercourse, or oral sex, or intercourse with ejaculation between the thighs, are all recognized methods of avoiding pregnancy. Some couples reserve vaginal intercourse for only the less fertile time of the menstrual cycle, and use a combination of mutual masturbation and other forms of non-genital sex for the rest of the time.

The second method of natural family planning is to avoid vaginal intercourse whenever pregnancy might occur, by making careful observations of the cyclical changes that occur in the body to try and predict the likeliest time for pregnancy. This is one of those things that is easy to do, but even easier to get wrong, and careful teaching is needed. The method relies on the fact that women usually ovulate about two weeks before menstruation, and are at their most fertile a few days before ovulation, when the mucus produced by the cervix is able to keep spermatozoa healthy and ready to meet the oocyte. Many women find that their temperature rises by about half a degree after ovulation, and so keeping careful records of the dates of periods, observing the changes that occur in the cervix and its mucus, and taking your temperature can tell you when to avoid intercourse and when it is safe to start again. The method works well for committed couples, but for those who are not well-taught or well-motivated there is a reputation for failure, which has given it the unfair nickname of 'Vatican roulette'.

The third method of natural family planning uses the

natural antifertility effect of breastfeeding. When women breastfeed the hormones produced by stimulation of the nipple affect or even prevent the development of oocytes. For most women there is a marginal reduction in fertility, but for those who feed frequently, on demand and for those whose infants the breast is the only source of nourishment, the contraceptive effect is profound. Breastfeeding is not an important contraceptive in Europe or North America, where women tend to feed their babies at regular set intervals, rather than frequently throughout the day and night, which reduces the frequency of nipple stimulation. They also supply other foods to their baby at an early stage, which has the same effect. However, this trend is changing and demand feeding is becoming more common in developed countries Breastfeeding is important in the context of the world's population, where a few years ago it was estimated that it was preventing more births than all the other methods of contraception put together. There is an obvious Catch 22; you have to have a baby before you can use this method of contraception.

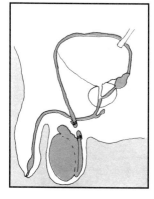

Male sterilization
The surgeon injects a drug to numb the skin over the scrotum, makes two small incisions on either side in it, and then cuts the vas deferens, which runs just below the skin. Occasionally a surgeon will also remove a piece of the vas. However, this is unnecessary, because a small cut in the right place is just as effective as removing a large chunk, but bigger operations can lead to other damage happening, as well as making reversal of the operation impossible should the man change his mind.

Sterilization

Not everybody wants a reversible method of contraception. For some people there are medical reasons not to have children whilst others feel that they never want to run the risk of a pregnancy interfering with their lifestyle, but the vast majority of couples who choose one of the permanent methods of birth control are those who have had one or two children, and no longer want to bother with contraceptives, and their risks, and the possibility of them failing. Either men or women can be sterilized.

Male sterilization: vasectomy
Sterilizing men is a simple procedure that can be performed without the need for a general anaesthetic to put you to sleep. Spermatozoa are still produced after a vasectomy, but cannot reach the outside, and so are broken down by the body, and their constituents recycled. Semen is still produced, by the prostate and other glands, and so

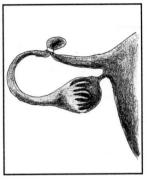

Female sterilization
Surgeons need to make a small cut - perhaps only a couple of centimetres long - through the skin and muscle of the front of the abdomen. Nowadays they block the fallopian tube with plastic clips or rings, although once there was a vogue for burning or electrically cauterizing the tubes. Few women stay in hospital for more than a few hours after the operation, and most resume normal life, perhaps feeling nothing more than a bit stiff and sore, the next day.

ejaculation and orgasm are unimpaired, but because there are still many spermatozoa downstream of the vasectomy site, men do not lose their fertility for some months after the operation. Most clinics check a man's semen two and three months after the operation and expect to find no spermatozoa at all then.

Female sterilization
In essence, female sterilization is the same as male sterilization: the tube carrying the gametes is divided. But, because the man's vas lies just under the skin, it is easy to divide and the whole procedure take a few minutes without the need for anything more than numbing of the skin.

The fallopian tube, however, is deep inside the abdomen, and most surgeons who sterilize women do so in hospital when the women are under a general anaesthetic.

Sterilization in women is effective immediately, but a little more likely to fail than vasectomy. After a successful vasectomy perhaps one man in 5000 will have an unexpected return of fertility, often many years after the operation, but after a female sterilization there is a chance that one woman in 200 will find herself pregnant. Men can have a simple test to see if they still have spermatozoa in their ejaculate; women have to wait and see if they conceive. One other problem with failure of sterilization in women is that the pregnancy that results may be in the fallopian tube because the attempt at blockage, or the body's attempts to overcome the blockage, leaves a small gap in the tube which allows spermatozoa through. This is an uncommon, but dangerous, complication.

Morning-after contraception
What do you do if you have an accident, a condom bursts, or is forgotten, and you think there is a risk you might become pregnant?

Nearly all family planning clinics, and most family doctors, now offer morning-after contraception. To be strictly accurate, it need not be the morning after - you can use something to prevent pregnancy for a week after intercourse, and with the new preparations that will be on the market in the next decade, even longer after an accident. But don't delay - get your treatment as soon as possible.

There are two methods available in Britain today. The first is to take four oral contraceptive pills. These are not the standard type of tablets that most women take, but a higher dose no longer widely used, but still safe. The four tablet dose is effective, and will prevent pregnancy in 98% of women who are at risk. The side-effects are few but include nausea, vomiting, breast tenderness and menstrual upsets. These are not, however, disabling. The tablets must be taken within 72 hours of intercourse. The morning-after pill works in several ways, but principally it blocks the specialized receptors in the endometrium that recognize hormones and are essential for successful implantation of the embryo.

The second method is to fit an intrauterine device. This needs to be done within a week of the accident. The IUD interferes directly with the endometrium and prevents the embryo implanting. As a method it is more effective than taking the tablets, in that less than one woman in 1000 who uses this will become pregnant, but there are some problems.

The first is that fitting an IUD is a skilled procedure and as the number of women using the IUD is falling, there are correspondingly fewer doctors experienced in fitting them especially in an emergency. Also, the IUD can make infections in the pelvis more severe, and if there is a possibility of infection from the person who also gave you the risk of pregnancy, the IUD can make matters much worse.

The IUD is also less easy to fit in the uterus of a woman who has had no children , and especially one who is young. Unfortunately, it is young women who are most at risk of sex without contraception, so the group who need help most are those who are least able to use the best method of morning-after contraception.

Abortion

Not every pregnancy is planned and wanted, and in societies

that do not make contraception (especially morning-after contraception) freely available, some women will become pregnant without wanting to. Neither Ireland nor the United States of America give all people (especially young people) easy access to contraception. In both countries more young women have unwanted pregnancies removed as abortions than in Britain. Conversely, morning-after contraception is widely advertised and discussed in The Netherlands, and proportionately fewer women have abortions there than in Sweden, where morning-after contraception is freely available, but hardly ever advertised or used.

In most of the world abortion is legal and openly available. Experience in many countries shows that restricting access to abortion makes women have criminal abortions, which are unsafe, whilst poorer women, who can usually cope less well with unwanted pregnancy, suffer. Abortion is more fully discussed in other textbooks (see the reading list at the end of this book), but in essence there are two main methods used.

The first is to remove the pregnancy by stretching the cervix, and sucking the contents from the uterus. This is done in early pregnancy, and is safe. It can be done under a general anaesthetic, or after numbing the cervix with local anaesthetic. Depending on the skill of the surgeon it is safe for the first third, or first half, of pregnancy.

For more advanced pregnancy, or where the surgeon feels unhappy about using this approach after the first third of pregnancy, the commonest technique is to give drugs to make the woman go into labour. These drugs can be injected into the uterus, around the uterus, into a vein, or placed in the vagina. After anything from an hour or two to a day or two the pregnancy is expelled.

Pregnancy

This book is not long enough to discuss the whole of pregnancy. There is a list of recommended books at the back; they have much more information for you.

For most women their sex life does not end because

they are pregnant, but it often changes, either because they feel uncomfortable as the baby grows, or because the changes in the hormone levels reduce or increase their desire, or they are concerned for the welfare of their baby. The latter problem arises because of the old wives' tales about the dangers of sex in pregnancy. The only possible danger arises with oral sex; if you blow into the vagina of a pregnant woman it is possible for air to enter the uterus, and the blood vessels behind the placenta which can be fatal for the fetus.

The menopause

The menopause marks the end of reproductive life for women, just as puberty marks the beginning. But the menopause is not a sign of senescence, simply another change in status.

The menopause is the ending of menstruation, the time when the last of the four million oocytes a woman was created are used up. One unfortunate consequence of this ending of ovulation is that no more oestrogen hormones are produced, and it is oestrogens that are responsible for keeping many of the tissues of the body healthy. These oestrogens can be replaced artificially; this is discussed in more specialized books mentioned in the reading list at the end of this book.

What does the menopause mean for your sex life? Mostly, it means good things. The fear of pregnancy, which can be inhibiting for many couples, disappears. The mood changes that are associated with menstruation also go. At about this time family responsibilities often also change, and this too can be of great benefit.

But there are some problems. The vulva and vagina are sensitive to oestrogens, and so without regular oestrogens from the ovary they sometimes shrink, and may even become painful during intercourse. Care, and lubrication, and sometimes oestrogen used either as a cream or in another fashion, are often all that is needed. If you have problems, call in and see your doctor early.

Maintaining sexual health

Keeping your sex life healthy is more than obeying the simple rules that keep the rest of your life healthy. Certainly, the most important way to maintain sexual health is to keep your general health standards high but you also need to acquire information, and the rest of this chapter will include simple health rules, and a clear discussion of some of the most important infections that affect sexual health. The descriptions of sexually transmitted infections are not meant to frighten you, but simply make you aware of the possible problems that can interfere with your enjoyment of sex.

Sexual health in men

Men need to exercise, and watch their diet. This is not just to make sure they are fit enough to enjoy themselves sexually. There are two more practical points to consider. The first is that in both men and women fat cells make some hormones, and change others into different forms. Men who are too fat have high levels of oestradiol, which is principally a female hormone. This additional hormone is both produced by fat cells, and converted by them using other hormones as building blocks. Oestradiol in low levels is normal, but in high levels in men depresses sexual desire, fertility, and sexual performance. It may also lead to heart and blood vessel disease, which is another problem both medically and sexually.

Problems with the heart and blood vessels follow on from being overweight and from getting insufficient exercise, and even more so from smoking cigarettes. And there are several important reasons for avoiding blood vessel disease. But before we consider the sexual side of such disease, some general aspects.

It may seem strange in a book such as this one, to write about a problem that only affects one system of the body, but because blood vessels supply every other part of the body with nutrients and oxygen, and take away waste products and carbon dioxide, anything that makes them work less effectively can have a damaging effect elsewhere.

Blood vessel disease is more common in men than women. The term is short-hand for several different conditions, but all start with damage to the membrane lining the inside of arteries and veins. After the damage there is furring of the arteries and to a lesser extent the veins, which make them less able to carry blood. Sometimes the blood vessel bursts, and if this happens in the brain the result is called a stroke. A sudden blockage in blood vessels supplying the heart results in a heart attack. More usually the amount of blood carried to the particular organ decreases slowly over a relatively long period of time, and the organ gradually loses function. This means that small nerves can be damaged before you notice the changes. (Large important structures usually have several blood vessels so that if one is damaged the others continue the blood supply.) And some of the more important small nerves are those that are responsible for starting, and maintaining, erections. Erection follows a delicate interaction of signals from the nerves and hormones that act on blood vessels. If the blood supply to the lower body is poor this can prevent erection from happening.

Sometimes one of the early signs of blood vessel disease is severe chest pain when you get excited. For one third of people the earliest sign is sudden death. This pain, called angina, can be crippling, and is a sign that the heart muscle is not getting enough oxygen. The way to prevent the pain when an attack occurs is to stop what you are doing and rest, which is tough if you are in the middle of making love.

There is another reason for watching your weight. Being overweight contributes to high blood pressure, and high blood pressure leads to blood vessel disease, which indirectly is the most important and commonest cause of death in men in the Western world. So doctors look for high blood pressure, and when they find men (or women) with it they treat it. But unfortunately, many of the drugs used to treat high blood pressure also reduce the ability of men to have erections, or affect their capacity for orgasm, or both.

Commonly used medicines can affect fertility, the

ability to have erections, and the capacity for sexual arousal. These drugs include diuretics such as frusemide, hydrochlorthiazide, ethacrynic acid, spironolactone; blood pressure treatments such as methyldopa and hydralazine; and ß-blockers such as propranolol, clonidine. Other drugs that have this effect include many of the tranquilizers and antidepressants used by psychiatrists. Some anti-histamines (used for the treatment of hay fever), and drugs used to treat gastric and duodenal ulcers have similar effects. Both cigarette smoking and drinking alcohol reduce fertility and, in the long-term, impair sexual performance through their effects on blood vessels and their direct toxic effects. Alcohol is an important cause of high blood pressure. Some sexually transmitted infections impair fertility, and all may have long-term effects that sometimes only become apparent many years after the initial problem.

Sexual health in women

The same rules apply to women, but there are two additional special circumstances, pregnancy and the menopause. In pregnancy there may be a reduction in sex drive, and the physical discomforts may also make sexual activity less pleasant. The menopause is characterized by a reduction in the amount of sex hormone produced, with pronounced effects on the genital organs, as well as the rest of the body and the psyche.

The consequences of pelvic infection are more serious in women than in men, and this is discussed later in this section. In most societies the burden of contraception falls more on women than on men, and so they need to understand the risks and benefits more than men do.

Sexually transmitted infections

Sexually transmitted infections are common, and important. Gonorrhoea is now commoner and as infectious in most Western countries as is measles, although this is partly because there are good vaccines against measles, which you can only catch once anyway.

Why are these infections so common? And why are they so important? To deal with the last question first. Any disease that interferes with sexual enjoyment should be treated, but the special importance of sexually transmitted disease is their seeming unimportance. Most of them appear to do little harm to most of the people who get them, and this has been true for centuries. Although syphilis has ravaged whole communities in the past, there was a time when even it was considered an acceptable condition for young men to acquire whilst sowing their wild oats.

But the situation has changed, because we now realize that many of the infections once considered trivial actually have more serious consequences, and that AIDS, which was once thought of as a disease resulting purely from anal intercourse, is now recognized as being much more than that, now that it has reached the heterosexual community. AIDS is probably always fatal, which means that catching the virus that causes it is potentially a death sentence. The alarm that AIDS has provoked is at last beginning to provoke rethinking about sexually transmitted disease, although because there is a shortage of information on the subject not all of that rethinking is as constructive as it could be.

Why are these infections so common?

All spread of sexually transmitted infections could be prevented for ever if each person only ever had one sexual partner for life. It is rather naive to think that this state will ever be achieved, and so we might as well be realistic and think about the world as it actually is, not as idealists would like it to be.

The risk for sexually transmitted disease comes from the fact that all people, and not just the young, are more mobile than their ancestors were. They expect to spend some time living and working away from home, they expect to go to other cities or other countries for their education, and they expect to go abroad for holidays, and if they are young, without their parents. All of these make casual sexual encounters more likely to occur. And since most of the infections described in the next few pages are

Society and STD

There are two ways of dealing with sexually transmitted disease. The first is to be punitive, and in some parts of the world men and women with sexually transmitted disease face prison sentences. Many armies used to court-martial soldiers found to have any form of sexually transmitted disease, on the grounds that treating them used up military resources, and made the men unfit for fighting whilst they were being cured. Military and civilian clinics in such societies reflected that sort of official attitude, which meant few people attended them, and tracing contacts was difficult. People were too ashamed to admit to new partners that they may have some form of infection, and so treatable diseases were ignored, and perhaps also spread because no one wanted to warn future partners.

Thankfully things have changed now. A much more modern approach is to be open, and treat sexually transmitted infections as any other. Clinics are friendlier, and more accessible, but still manage to preserve confidentiality.

not obvious for many of those who have them, people unwittingly spread disease.

In Britain, prostitution is not important as a cause of sexually transmitted disease in the rest of the population, although there is some argument about the definition of the word. Most women whose principal income comes from selling sexual favours know how to look after their bodies. They are usually selective about with whom they have sex, and they usually insist on their customers using condoms. Condoms do not eliminate the risk of sexually transmitted infection, but they reduce it.

There is another group of women who are a greater source of concern. They are inadequate socially, often unemployed, and drift from man to man in a disorganized way, and sometimes support themselves and their partner by additional prostitution. They may be more of a risk to others for sexually transmitted infections than those working principally as prostitutes, but in general, it is the enthusiastic amateur, both male and female, who is at greatest risk of giving and receiving infections.

AIDS is a special case. AIDS can be spread through blood, and in some cities the biggest reservoir of AIDS are those who misuse drugs. Some addicts support themselves and their partners and their drug habits by prostitution, and they are often too disorganized to use condoms reliably. And perhaps, some of those who have AIDS, or are drug addicts, don't care what happens to other people any more.

Controlling the spread

The infections now being described are spread sexually. Most of the organisms are remarkably delicate, and die when they get dry, or exposed to light or sunshine, and so you won't get them from lavatory seats, or eating food cooked by someone with them. You get them when a warm and moist part of your body comes into contact with a warm and moist part of someone else's. So you need to think about your partners, and what you do with them, and what they do with other people. There are lots of very nice well-brought-up men and women, who only ever have one sexual partner between birth and death, who get sexually transmitted infections. They get them because either their partner had such an infection when they first met, or acquired it later. Perhaps that is why sexually transmitted disease arouses such emotions: there is a strong element of betrayal.

So people need to do more than ask about infections. They need additional protection. One obvious form of protection is to make sure that you and your partner have never had other partners, and will never have other partners, but as we said at the beginning, that is a pious hope. The next best thing to do is be selective about your partners, but even here things are difficult. There is little point in saying that you should never have sex with someone whom you are unlikely to meet again; as we said at the beginning of this section, it is precisely because so many people are prepared to take this risk that there is a problem in the first place. Holiday romances are notorious for ending in tears.

At a more practical level, avoid risks by using barrier contraceptives. The condom is not a perfect device; it was once described by a French woman as 'Armour against love, but gossamer against infection'. But at least it is better than nothing. And contraceptive creams and foams kill not only spermatozoa, but also many of the bacteria, viruses, and other parasites that cause sexually transmitted diseases.

But, barrier contraceptives can be a humiliating thing to insist on. If you ask your new partner to use a condom, you are perhaps implying that either you think he is infected, or you know you are. It is hard, but you need to face up to that point, and if you are unwilling to do so, then you are probably better off not taking the risk.

There are good evolutionary instincts that make people careless about contraception; if everybody used contraception every time they made love, the human race would die out. You are using contraception in this instance not to thwart evolutionary forces, but to improve the quality of your life.

The next practical step is to make use of one of the

How can we prevent the spread of sexually transmitted disease?

The first thing to do is to be open about the problem. That is difficult; it is hard enough to broach the subject of sex with a new partner, but to go on from there to talk about contraception, and then ask about diseases in their past ... Even that is not enough.

From page 47 to 57 most of the common sexually transmitted diseases are discussed, but they are written about from a medical point of view. They are described as diseases, but remember that for most of them, men and women who have them will be unaware that they are infected. It may be because they are still incubating the disease, but much more likely they have no symptoms, yet are still infectious. It is possible for someone to acquire an infection, pass it on to a second partner, who gives it to a third, and only the fourth will have symptoms.

Special clinics

The routine depends a lot on the clinic you go to. You may have to make an appointment, or it may be a walk-in service. You will get the chance to see a skilled doctor of the same sex as yourself, and you will probably also see a nurse. You will find that they are sympathetic, and are unlikely to be shocked by anything you tell them. They will ask about your fears and worries, and the symptom (if there is one) that prompted you to come to the clinic. They will usually take blood from you, examine you, and take smears and swabs with which to look for bacteria from your genitals. Some people are upset by the many swabs that are taken from several different sites. This is done so that there is little chance of missing any infection. Most clinics will retest you a few weeks later, and if they find anything amiss will always retest you after treatment to make sure that there is nothing to worry about. The clinic staff will try and trace your contacts, or help you to trace them; you will also have the opportunity of discussing problems such as contraception, and ways of reducing your risks in the future.

special clinics for sexually transmitted disease if you have any concerns about your sexual health, or a recent encounter. Almost every medium sized town has such a clinic, and certainly every big city has at least one. If you feel too embarrassed to use the one in your home town, then go to the nearest anonymous big city and visit a clinic there.

Don't just use these clinics when you have a problem; go there if you think you have taken a risk. You need not worry about the skill of the staff, or their attitude to confidentiality. In Britain the law is strict about the qualifications of those who work in clinics for sexually transmitted disease, because parliament recognizes that the fears and embarrassments of shy people leave them open to exploitation. If you go to a reputable clinic you will get first class service. If you go to somewhere other than a recognized sexually transmitted disease clinic, such as some family planning clinics, you will probably still get a first class service, but the people working there would be the first to admit that they have none of the sophisticated equipment for making a diagnosis that is found in the specialized clinics. So don't take chances with your health.

The last important step in reducing the incidence of infection is contact tracing. This is a specialized skill. It happens after a definite diagnosis of one of the sexually transmitted diseases has been made. It involves a counsellor talking with you, and trying to find out about the person who infected you, and those whom you in turn might have infected. It can be a deeply upsetting interview, but the contact tracers are all skilled and caring people, and they do a great job.

What diseases are sexually transmitted?

There are dozens of diseases capable of being spread sexually, but this section will concentrate on the most important.

The availability of cheap air travel and the popularity of holidays abroad have increased the problem for clinic staff, because diseases that were once rare, or limited to sailors on board ships that went to the tropics, can now be found in the most unlikely cities. Similarly, since inadequate treatment of infections of any type can lead to the organism being not destroyed, but simply becoming resistant to the antibiotic, poor health standards in some parts of the world mean that specialists in other countries are finding their work made difficult.

Not every vaginal infection is sexually transmitted, although for convenience all important vaginal infections are described in this section. The vagina is warm and moist, and would normally be expected to be an ideal breeding ground for all sorts of infection. It is not, because there are several natural factors that prevent infection. One is that the vagina is acidic, and kept that way by the bacteria that live there. The cells are also tough, and well-adapted to their function.

Several things increase the likelihood of vaginal infection. The lubricating fluid produced when a women is aroused neutralizes the acid, as does semen. So intercourse too frequently, or with too many men, can alter the vaginal environment, and make infection more likely. Vaginal douching washes out the normal bacteria, and again makes infection more likely. After the menopause the vagina becomes thinner, and less able to resist infection.

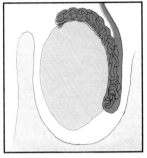

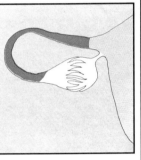

Gonorrhoea
Most women with gonorrhoea have no symptoms, although some get pain or swelling in the vulva a few days after they are first infected. Gonorrhoea commonly infects the urethra as well as the anus, and in both men and women it can spread deeper into the pelvis, giving an infection of the epididymis in men (top) which can make them sterile and of the fallopian tubes in women (below) which may also cause sterility.

Gonorrhoea

Along with syphilis (see page 51) gonorrhoea is probably the best known of all the sexually transmitted diseases. Syphilis is rare in Europe now, whilst gonorrhoea is common. Gonorrhoea is caused by a particular bacterium called the gonococcus. Injections of penicillin are used to treat the infection, but the misuse of penicillin in many parts of the world means that many cases of gonorrhoea are now caused by organisms that are resistant to penicillin, so it is not always a reliable treatment.

Thrush

Thrush is probably the commonest vaginal infection. It is not usually sexually transmitted, although it can be. It is caused by the organism *Candida albicans,* which is a form

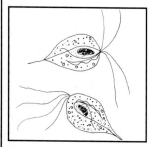

Trichomoniasis protozoan

of yeast. This yeast is present in and on all of us, all the time. Normally it is controlled by the effects of other organisms and the immune mechanisms of the body. But there are times when it gets out of control. This can happen during pregnancy, or treatment with antibiotics that might destroy the organisms that normally control the yeast, or treatment with other drugs that either affect those bacteria or the body's immune system. It can also happen in diabetes. This is a problem because diabetes leads to high levels of glucose in the urine, and in the cells of the vagina. The thrush yeast thrives in those conditions, and the control bacteria do not. There is one other social factor that increases the incidence of thrush. Nylon underwear makes it difficult for natural secretions to be drained away, as do other forms of tight clothing. Tight jeans, nylon tights, and similar items of clothing all make thrush more likely to happen. Thrush is not usually sexually transmitted, but there are exceptions.

The variety of thrush that most of us have on or in our bodies is harmless. The variety that causes infections is different. It has usually evolved from the benign form in the woman (or man) who has it, but occasionally it can be sexually acquired. It can also ping-pong between partners, and so if they both have the organism, and only one is treated at a time, then the cleared partner can keep getting reinfected by the other. Treatment is simple. There is a wide variety of drugs that will kill the yeast, and it is worth trying several if the first does not work.

Prevention is much better. Don't wear nylon! Wear cotton pants, loose clothes, and stockings rather than tights. And when you do not need to, don't wear underwear at all. There is nothing wrong with that, especially at home. Change the way you live. Don't sit in hot baths. Cut out sugar and chocolate from your diet. Alcohol can make thrush worse, or make it become obvious for the first time. If you keep getting the disease, see a specialist, and if you have a partner, get him or her treated as well.

Trichomoniasis
This is the second most common vaginal infection. It is

caused by a protozoan much larger than either bacteria or viruses. This parasite lives in glands around the urethra of both men and women, and it thrives in semen. It is one of the few organisms able to cause sexually transmitted infections that is not delicate; it has been known to survive for over a day in chlorinated swimming pool water, although by and large it is only sexually transmitted. The organism causes an itchy vaginal or penile discharge which is usually grey-white and can be frothy. It is treated with the antibiotic metronidazole which interacts with alcohol, making people who mix the two get nauseated.

Hepatitis

This is inflammation of the liver and there are two varieties, A and B. Hepatitis B is preventable by active vaccination, unlike Hepatitis A, which is more common in the UK, and can only be protected against using gamma-globulin.

Hepatitis B does not affect your sex life, but it can be sexually transmitted, which is why it is included here. The virus is usually spread through contact with blood or semen, or faeces, and so can be spread sexually. When the liver is infected the body can no longer cope with the break-down products that the liver normally deals with, and so the most obvious sign of illness is jaundice, when the skin turns yellow because of an excess of blood-cell pigments. Hepatitis is important because it can be fatal.

Gardnerella

There has been much discussion over this organism. It is difficult to culture in laboratories, which has accounted for part of the confusion.

Women with a vaginal infection caused by *Gardnerella vaginalis* have a thin, watery, opaque vaginal discharge with an unpleasant smell rather reminiscent of dead fish. This is especially noticeable after intercourse, because it seems that products of the organism interact with semen. The infection is easily treated with antibiotics, and does not seem to cause any long-term harm.

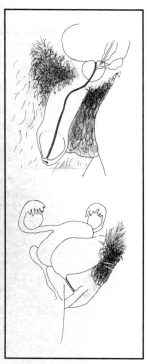

Cystitis is more common in women, who have a shorter urethra than men.

Salpingitis

Salpingitis is infection of the fallopian tube. It is almost always sexually acquired, but can follow the insertion of an IUD, or gynaecological surgery.

It is a serious disease, usually requiring admission to hospital, and can have serious consequences. The fallopian tubes are delicate organs, and when damaged can either fail to function, so that the affected woman becomes infertile, or be partially damaged, and so predispose to ectopic pregnancy (pregnancy in the fallopian tube).

The disease can follow an infection in the cervix or vagina, or it can follow intercourse when infected spermatozoa carry bacteria on their outer surface. (Spermatozoa are designed to penetrate as far as the fallopian tubes.)

Bacteria are prevented from entering the body by cervical mucus, the antibodies produced in it and by the endometrium. Menstrual blood is alkaline, and so salpingitis is more likely to occur in the few days after menstruation, when the acid vagina has been neutralized by the menstrual blood, the uterine cavity is raw because the endometrium has just been shed, and the cervical mucus has also been washed away.

Salpingitis is treated with antibiotics, sometimes injected directly into a vein to make sure that high concentrations reach the fallopian tubes.

Cystitis

Cystitis is common, and rarely sexually transmitted, although at the same time cystitis is rare in women who do not have intercourse.

Cystitis simply means inflammation of the bladder. It is characterized by pain when you pass urine, sometimes passing blood in your urine, and a desire to urinate more frequently than usual.

It is rare in men, and common in women for a number of reasons. Men have a long urethra, and so it is difficult for the bacteria to get from the outside through to the bladder. The prostate produces natural antibiotics that kill bacteria before they get to the bladder. Women, however, have a short urethra which is close to the anus, and can be easily bruised during intercourse. This bruising can produce the symptoms of cystitis.

When doctors cannot find a bacterial cause of cystitis, it is possible that the woman does not have a bladder infection but simply has pain in her urethra because of sex.

Syphilis

Syphilis is not a common disease in Britain. It was once the most important of all the sexually transmitted diseases. It is referred to as 'the pox' in many of Shakespeare's plays, because in late syphilis the skin breaks out in many pocks, which do not heal easily (especially true in the days before penicillin).

Syphilis, in its early stages, appears to cure itself, but if left untreated it silently progresses to a more serious disease that can affect almost every other system in the body.

The disease starts as a small, shallow ulcer which is painless, and may be unnoticed if it is on an inner surface of the body. The incubation period is between one and twelve weeks, although for most people it is between two and four weeks. The ulcer heals, and then between six weeks and two years later there is often a skin rash, which can mimic almost every known skin disease. The rash is usually wide-spread, and disappears after a short time.

Syphilis then enters the latent phase. It can disappear completely, or progress to damage the heart, blood vessels, brain or any other body system. If the disease progresses it is usually with serious consequences. Because some of the men and women who get syphilitic disease of the brain end up in mental hospitals, there is a tradition that any politician, especially a foreign one, who behaves in a despotic fashion is said to be suffering from the late stages of syphilis. This has been said of individuals such as Idi Amin, Adolf Hitler and King Henry VIII, with no proof in any case.

Pregnant women with syphilis can infect their unborn children. The consequences for the child are devastating, and in most countries of the world every pregnant woman is automatically screened for syphilis during preg-

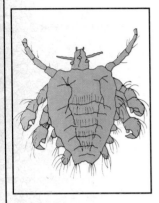

Crabs

Crabs are common, and rarely serious. These particular crabs are small insects, more properly called the crab lice, which have only a passing resemblance to the animals you find in the sea. They are tiny and have six long legs, designed to hang onto hair. The pubic louse is different from those that survive on general body hair or the scalp. The louse is blood-sucking and is usually passed on sexually, but can be acquired from infected bed clothes. Since it is spread from pubic hair to pubic hair, using condoms does not help prevent the spread.
The infection is treated with an insecticidal shampoo.

nancy, usually without her knowledge. It is rare for a test to be positive, and even rarer for it to be due to syphilis, (because many other diseases give false-positive results). Treatment with penicillin is usually effective.

The search for a cure for syphilis led to some of the most intensive medical research before the 'magic bullet' that would destroy syphilis but not the patient was found. Early treatments were based on arsenic, but penicillin is now the standard.

Chlamydia

Most people infected with chlamydia probably have no symptoms, but it can lead to a wide variety of problems. It affects the mucosa of the bladder and urethra (causing urethritis) in both men and women, leading to pain when passing urine. This is similar to the pain caused by infection with the gonorrhoea bacterium, and it is possible that many of the problems that were once diagnosed as post-gonococcal urethritis, or non-gonococcal urethritis, were actually caused by chlamydia.

The organism also affects the rest of the pelvis in both men and women. Men can get a painful infection of the epididymis and testis, which can lead to infertility in later years. Women are more likely to suffer an infection of the cervix. This is of no consequence to the woman, but since she will probably be unaware of it, she can pass on the disease.

More seriously, the fallopian tube can be infected. Infection of the fallopian tube (salpingitis) leads to infertility, chronic pelvic pain, and the damaged fallopian tube can lead to ectopic pregnancy. Ectopic pregnancy occurs in about one per cent of all pregnancies (although most do not follow chlamydial infection) and can be treated only by an emergency operation, which usually results in the loss of that fallopian tube. If not treated it can be fatal, due to loss of blood.

Clamydia infection can spread beyond the pelvis. Infection of the area around the liver and gall bladder is characteristic of chlamydial infection, and scar tissue can develop at the site of this infection. There is also an uncommon complication of chlamydial infection known as Reiter's syndrome. This disease is probably an abnormal response to infection with the organism in people genetically predisposed to it, and is characterized by arthritis (pain in the joints, particularly the ankle), conjunctivitis (pain and inflammation in the eye) and urethritis. There are also skin rashes, and often ulcers on the penis. However, Reiter's syndrome may also have other causes. There have been suggestions, difficult to prove, that infection with chlamydia in pregnancy may predispose to losing that pregnancy.

Chlamydial infections are treated with antibiotics, for at least one week, and perhaps longer. Simple, safe, broad-spectrum antibiotics such as tetracycline and erythromycin, are effective.

It is difficult to eliminate the organism completely, and it is quite possible that in women it remains in the pelvis as a low-level infection for many years, and flares up when her resistance is low.

Herpes

The herpes virus family causes many diseases in humans. The commonest is the simple cold sore, but chickenpox and glandular fever all belong to this family. The most relevant to this section is genital herpes, which is caused by a variant of the herpes simplex virus (HSV), which normally causes the cold sore. Genital herpes is now extremely common, and there has been a ten-fold increase in the estimated number of people who have contracted it over the past decade.

Genital herpes is caused by the Type II strain of the virus, usually abbreviated to HSVII or HSV2. HSVI was once thought to cause cold sores around the mouth and HSVII was thought to be restricted to the genitals, but the increasing frequency of oral sex has made the difference meaningless. The only practical point is that people who have antibodies to one type, perhaps from a cold sore when they were young, tend to get a less severe form of genital herpes.

After catching the virus there is an incubation period

Seventy years ago two German specialists described a particular type of cell in the pus from eyes of new-born babies with conjunctivitis and also in the cells from the cervix of the mothers. With hindsight it is obvious that they were describing a sexually transmitted infection that the mothers were passing on to their infants, but it took a long time for the link to be made, and for it to be realized that the problem was caused by the Chlamydia trachomatis organism. This is a parasite that lies mid-way between bacteria and viruses in complexity. It is related to the organism that causes psittacosis, a disease that affects humans and parrots. Chlamydia is difficult to culture in the laboratory, which is part of the explanation for the long time it took the medical profession to realize how important it was, and also how common.

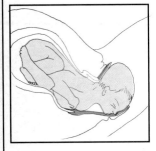

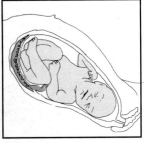

Two things may happen if the woman is pregnant when she has her first attack of herpes. The first is that the virus may cross the placenta (above) and damage the baby by overwhelming infection. The second is that the baby may be infected as it passes through the vagina during birth (below). In either case the infection rapidly spreads, and the baby, who has no defence against it, may either die, or if it survives, be severely handicapped because of herpes virus infection of the brain.

of three to six days, during which the person is usually quite well, but may have a fever, or headache, or some other signs of illness.

The rash appears over the genitals as a crop of blisters that soon burst to leave small, extremely painful, ulcers. These heal rapidly, and there is rarely any scarring. The rash is present for about two weeks, and heals in about four. However, the disease never quite goes away, and there is a potential effect on pregnancy.

After the original infection the virus retires to hide in local nerves and may stay there unnoticed for decades. Or it may flare up a few days after the first attack. Each attack can be as unpleasant and painful as the first, and generally appears without warning, often when the person is under stress, but usually without predisposing factors. Women are more likely to get recurrent attacks at about the time of menstruation. There is a tendency for the attacks to get less frequent and less severe as the person ages, but this might not be for many years. Recurrent attacks are often preceded by about 24-72 hours of feeling unwell, and then clear up in about 8-14 days.

The potential effect on pregnancy caused much anxiety a few years ago. Fortunately the first attack is the only one to cause problems in pregnancy: subsequent attacks cause pain to the woman, but do not affect her pregnancy in any way.

All of this is uncommon, and applies to a first attack late in pregnancy, which is also uncommon. If you have had herpes in the past, you can become pregnant safely. You will not need a Caesarean section to prevent your baby picking up the infection during birth.

Treatment has changed over the past decade. At one stage doctors could prescribe only painkilling drugs or ointments, and antibiotics to stop other bacteria infecting the ulcers. But there are now drugs that act specifically against the virus, stopping its spread. This may make subsequent recurrences less likely to occur, and shorten the time the victim is unwell. There is still no vaccine to prevent the disease, although scientists are working on it.

54

Genital warts

Genital warts have been known about for millennia. Early in the second century the physician Soranus wrote a treatise entitled 'On Warty Excrescences in the Female Genitalia'. Unfortunately it was almost 2000 years before medical scientists took much interest in them again. In the 1890s scientists realized that genital warts were infectious: they gave volunteers skin warts by injecting extracts of warts from one man's penis into another's skin. Not much more research was done in the next few decades; it was felt that genital warts were simply skin warts in a different site, and not particularly related to sexual activity.

Once again, war helped doctors study this sexually transmitted disease. American scientists studied servicemen returning from the Korean war. They knew when the men had acquired their wart infection, and by studying the time it took for warts to appear on the men's wives, they were able to determine that genital warts were sexually transmitted, with an incubation period of about four to six weeks.

Genital warts

Genital warts are now recognized as being very common and perhaps one woman in five who is sexually active has some sign of the virus. Because warts do not cause many symptoms they are becoming commoner; most people do not ask their doctors about problems they are not aware of.

The warts are caused by a small DNA tumour virus. There is a whole family of these viruses, with many dozens of members, called the human papilloma virus (HPV). The most important ones from the point of view of human medicine are HPV16 and HPV18, because these are associated with cancers. The cervical inflammation associated with HPV6 and HPV11 rarely progress to cancer.

The HPV is important because this virus may sometimes have the ability to become malignant, in other words, to change the cells they have infected into cancerous cells. This is important to both sexes. In areas of the world where cancer of the penis is common (for example, in Uganda where it is the commonest cancer found in men) the possible cause is infection with a particular HPV. The virus may also be part of the reason that anal cancer is more common among homosexual men than heterosexual men.

In Europe the main importance of the virus is the possible link with cancers of the cervix, vulva and vagina. The last two cancers are relatively uncommon, but cancer of the cervix is an important cause of disease and death. The wart virus on its own is unlikely to cause cancer; it needs a co-carcinogen, which is a compound that acts together with another to cause cancer. The most powerful co-carcinogen freely available in Europe is cigarette tar, which probably explains the increased incidence of these cancers in cigarette smokers, or those who live with them. It is not known what the co-carcinogen that causes cancer of the penis is in Uganda.

Genital warts do not look like warts in other parts of the body. They are usually found in the moister areas, and they are soft pinky-white growths that look as if they have multiple small branches or fingers sticking out. They occur particularly in areas exposed to friction during intercourse.

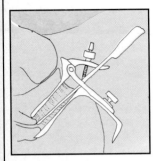

Severe inflammation of the cervix is easily and successfully treated by cervical cautery which removes the pre-cancerous tissue and prevents it spreading any further.

There is no perfect treatment for genital warts. Several drugs that act against viruses are being tried, but most clinics simply burn them off, either with a laser or with caustic chemicals. Once they have been burnt off they often regrow, but a second or third attempt at treatment is usually sufficient to keep them away. Women who have had warts, especially those who smoke, should have regular cervical smears for the rest of their lives.

Cancer of the cervix

Cancer of the cervix is not a sexually transmitted disease, but sometimes behaves as if were one. There are two kinds, and the common form, the one we usually mean when we talk about cervical cancer, is rare in women who have never had intercourse, but commoner amongst those who have had other sexually transmitted infections. The actual cause is unknown, but it seems to be linked to infection with the human papilloma virus (see page 55).

The cancer can be treated by surgery, radiotherapy, or, in the late stages, relieved by drugs, but prevention and early detection are much better. Prevent the disease by using barrier contraceptives and being careful in your choice of partner. Have regular cervical smears so that early changes can be detected. Treatment at this stage is successful and permanent.

AIDS

It is impossible to write anything on sex today without mentioning AIDS. AIDS - the Acquired Immune Deficiency Syndrome - is a new disease that can be spread sexually, or through infected blood. It is spread by a virus, the HIV or Human Immunodeficiency Virus.

This virus infects the body, and spreads to the cells of the immune system, destroying the capability of the body to respond to infection. It can cause some rare cancers, such as Kaposi's sarcoma, and give them a more rapid course. It can also spread to the brain, leading to a form of dementia.

Most people with AIDS die from infections, and

usually from unusual infections. The disease was first noticed when young healthy men began dying of previously obscure pneumonias, or got thrush so badly that instead of simply having a rash they were dying of thrush in the bloodstream. In the early days men who died were all homosexual; they were at especial risk because then young homosexual men were remarkably sexually active, with a great many different partners. This made them vulnerable to sexually transmitted infections, especially one such as AIDS with a latent phase after infection of several years, during which time the victims were infectious, but symptom-free.

AIDS is perhaps a good example of control of sexually transmitted disease. When it first became apparent there was hysteria, but there was less concern when it seemed to be restricted to the homosexual community; many people had a 'serve them right' attitude. There was neither the knowledge nor the desire to prevent it. The organized homosexual community in the United States and Europe responded by promoting the idea of safe sex, and this seems to have reduced the incidence of infection amongst them. Unhappily, it has not had the same effect on either the Third World, where AIDS is becoming more common, or the young, who are resistant to the ideas involved in health promotion, and often go through an experimental stage, where safe sex is not used because to do so would acknowledge that they were at risk.

Safer sex is any sexual activity that does not involve penetration or the exchange of body fluids, and so is considered risk-free. Most sexually transmitted diseases are infectious before they are apparent, and in the case of AIDS the interval between acquiring the disease, and being obviously ill with it may be five years, or even longer. Other diseases, such as infection with the chlamydia organism, may never lead to symptoms in many of the men and women who contract it, despite affecting their future health. Cancer of the cervix (the neck of the womb) may result from an infection, and 'safer sex' may prevent it. So if you want to be safe:
- *Be careful with your choice of partner.*
- *Avoid anything intimate until you are ready to commit yourself to him or her.*
- *Use barriers, especially with spermicides, and use them all the time.*

Avoidable conditions

Many of the conditions that cause sexual unhappiness are preventable, and most of those that are not are easily treated. This section is about keeping your sex life as healthy as possible, and where problems occur, treating them as soon as possible. It is an important area, because relationships that are purely sexual tend not to be long-lasting, but sexual discontent can spoil otherwise close partnerships.

The most important avoidable conditions have already been mentioned. Sexually transmitted diseases are common, and can be avoided, and with the exception of AIDS, readily and easily treated. Pregnancy can be avoided with simple, safe and effective contraception, and most types of infertility can be alleviated or circumvented. The menopause might not be avoidable, but many of the consequences of it are, and this is discussed in this section.

That leaves a few more specific areas of worry, and the bulk of this section discusses the treatment of sexual difficulties. Prevention of these is more difficult. Psychologists and educationalists have many theories about the correct way to bring up children to prevent them from developing irrational fears, dislikes and worries, whether about sex or anything else, but there is no proof that sexual problems develop from poor upbringing, or can be prevented by better education and teaching. What is obvious to those who work in this field is the importance of simple teaching for many people with sexual problems, and how a little learning, far from being dangerous, is of enormous help. The other important point to be made is that there is no substitute for both men and women understanding their partners.

Prevention of sexual difficulties

The most important avoidable conditions are lack of understanding and, closely associated with it, lack of knowledge. The only way of treating both of these is information. Not understanding basic physiology and the way people work may lead to unwarranted fears, as well as pregnancy, sexually transmitted disease, and unhappiness. Unfortunately, there are still many myths around about sex and sexuality, and men and women feel that if they don't live up to a stereotypical behaviour, they have a problem. But happiness does not depend on an understanding of physiology. You don't need a text-book to communicate with your partner. Just talk to him or her. And even more important - listen.

How common are sexual problems?

Some subjects are easy to study. We know how many children in Britain get polio every year because it is a rare disease, requires admission to hospital, and all cases of it are notified to the authorities. We can make an estimate of the number of people who get common colds every year; there are more of them, and even though the common cold is not a notifiable disease, estimates of its prevalence exist. But sexual problems are much harder to study. Many people with them do not go and see their doctor, and when they do, they often deny that the main reason for visiting the surgery is a problem with their sex life.

Sexual problems are relatively normal at some stages of life; for example, most men have difficulty in getting aroused when they are ill with a bad dose of influenza, and many women feel little sexual desire in the late stages of pregnancy. Many single men and women do not have a partner with whom to discover their sexual problem, although sometimes it is a real or imagined difficulty that is keeping them single.

But some studies have been done. Interpreting these is fraught with difficulty. People lie when given questionnaires, they feel embarrassed when interviewed, and they are much more likely to decline to take part in a survey of sexual matters than one of blood pressure, or of political opinions.

The first scientific studies were carried out in the United States in the decade beginning 1938 by Kinsey and his colleagues. Their work can be criticized as being old-fashioned and unrepresentative, but it pioneered much of the work now quoted. It also showed that some of the problems now regarded as new were common then.

The Kinsey studies contained no record of the proportion of men and women who lacked sexual interest, and no recognition of problems such as premature ejaculation. They showed that the proportion of men unable to have intercourse rose exponentially with age, whilst the proportion of women who had not achieved orgasm declined with age and experience. They also found that almost 13% of married women had never had an orgasm.

Other studies have used different methods of survey. One interesting study in the United States reported that whilst many women were aware of the sexual problems their husbands had, few men were aware of the difficulties their wives were experiencing. But all research has shown that sexual problems are common, in some studies affecting more than half of those sampled, probably more common in women than men, and that most people with such a problem want help, but do not know where to find it, and are often pessimistic about the outcome of such help. The reason for the finding that sexual problems seem to be more common in women may be a real difference, or it may simply reflect the fact that women are more likely than men to admit to such difficulties, since most men are trained from babyhood to be confident and deny the existence of personal problems, and women are more used to discussing sexual matters with gynaecologists and family planning clinic doctors.

Homosexuality

At least one problem of the past has now disappeared. Few people believe any more that homosexuality (sexual attraction to someone of the same sex) is a disease , but it may create a number of problems for people. Homosexuality has probably been practised since the first men and women formed the first social groups, and although no one knows for sure, it is probably no more common now than it was then. In some societies it has been the norm for young men and women to go through a homosexual stage before heterosexual relationships, and some armies, such as that of Sparta, encouraged homosexual love between soldiers to meld them into one fighting force.

Homosexuals are not men and women trapped into

a body of the 'wrong' sex; they recognize themselves for the sex that they are, and simply find their own sex more sexually attractive than the opposite sex. Homosexuality is unlikely to be caused entirely by either genetic or environmental factors; most homosexual men and women have heterosexual parents, went to heterosexual schools to be taught by heterosexual teachers, and have often spent some years living apparently normal heterosexual lives. Harmful traits tend to be bred out of society, and since homosexuals tend to have fewer children than heterosexuals, if homosexuality was harmful it should have disappeared by now. So the logical assumption is that it is a benign difference from the heterosexual norm of society. The other point to make is that homosexual men are no more effeminate than heterosexual men, and homosexual women are no more masculine than heterosexual women. Homosexuals do not form into partnerships where one acts out the role of a man and the other the women; if there are active and passive roles in homosexual intercourse then partners often swap.

Sexual problems

Older text books generally mention only two sexual problems; frigidity and impotence. Neither term is used by professionals nowadays, because they are too vague, and both have overtones of inadequacy and failure. There are also some sexual problems that relate to other important difficulties. As an example, for some couples fear of pregnancy affects the ability to enjoy intercourse, whilst for others the inability to conceive has a similarly depressing effect.

Female sexual problems

Modern thinking divides female sexual problems into impaired sexual interest, impaired sexual arousal, orgasmic dysfunction, vaginismus, dyspareunia, and sexual phobias. These are long words for fairly simple concepts. 'Dysfunction' simply means 'not functioning normally', and 'dyspareunia' means 'painful intercourse'.

Impaired sexual interest

This is probably the commonest problem seen in women. There is a wide range of features, from women uninterested in anything that any person does, to those who feel unable to respond to their principal partners but respond normally to other people, and those unable to initiate any form of sexual activity with their partner, but who respond once he or she has taken the initiative, and are then able to go on and experience arousal and orgasm.

The problem can be related simply to the woman's current partner or affect all her sexual relationships, and it can be present from her first experience of sex or from an unhappy experience with one person, or one experience with that person or something separate such as childbirth or bereavement. Depression can show itself as sexual difficulty.

Impaired sexual arousal

In this situation the normal responses described on pages 23-25 do not occur; there is reduced lubrication and lack of normal sexual sensations. This can be a feature of women with impaired sexual interest, or it can be a normal hormonal response to the changes associated with lack of ovulation, breastfeeding, and the menopause.

Orgasmic dysfunction

Many women have unrealistic expectations of the orgasm, and feel that if they do not experience several dozen one after the other, each one of which is able to make the earth move, then either they or their partner is inadequate. Other women are in the opposite situation; they have never experienced orgasm, and do not really care. There is a famous cartoon of such a woman drudging in the kitchen, who on being asked by a child reading a book 'Mummy, what's an orgasm?' replies 'Dunno, love, ask your father'. Some women have never climaxed, but this group is becoming smaller, because of sexual self-help books that provide simple instructions to help women grow to orgasm. Others do not achieve orgasm following vaginal intercourse, usually because their partner has provided insufficient stimulation. This might be because he has premature ejaculation, and tries desperately hard to keep his erection long enough to achieve intravaginal ejaculation, by avoiding any form of foreplay in case he becomes too excited, and ejaculates before entering the vagina. Other couples, often where there is a difficulty with the relationship, abandon foreplay because they want to get everything over with as soon as possible. This type of relationship difficulty can follow treatment for infertility, where sex has been devalued to something simply done on instructions from the clinic.

Vaginismus

The vaginal muscles are powerful, and not always under the direct control of the woman; involuntary tightening of them occurs. There are many lovely stories, all sworn to be true by a friend of someone in the pub, or another equally unlikely source, but all untrue, of the vaginal muscles clamping so tight during intercourse that the couple were unable to part. This cannot happen. What does happen is that the vaginal muscles clamp together so tightly that vaginal penetration cannot occur. This might be sufficient to prevent intercourse or the use of tampons.

Vaginismus can follow a vaginal infection, or poorly repaired surgery after childbirth. Or it can follow a painful condition that has healed, such that the expectation of a painful attempt at penetration makes the muscles go into spasm. And muscles that are in spasm hurt (think back to the last time you sprained your back or your ankle; the pain there was usually caused by muscular spasm). It can also be mimicked by something such as a tough hymen that cannot be ruptured, although this is uncommon.

Much more commonly, vaginismus follows specific sexual phobias or fantasies, that may have resulted from an unpleasant incident. A woman whose first attempt at vaginal penetration occurred when she was raped, or was a painful unpleasant experience that happened before she was fully aroused, is unlikely to look forward to the next attempt. Poor education also encourages vaginismus to develop. Women who are taught that the vagina is dirty, or that sex is part of the punishment women have to bear for the sins of Eve in the Garden of Eden, or that the vagina is tiny and the penis a huge organ that tears its way in, are unlikely to enjoy the thought of penetration, and so muscular spasm develops. This leads to pain and unpleasantness, and so becomes a self-fulfilling prophecy.

Vaginismus can also develop as the presenting problem for a woman whose main problem is lack of interest in either sex or sexual relations with her partner. Nobody believes now that women with vaginismus are secretly homosexual.

Dyspareunia, or painful intercourse
One survey suggested that 40% of women attending a gynaecology clinic had pain on intercourse, or when they used tampons. It is one of the commonest symptoms for which women seek gynaecological help.

The pain may be deep within the pelvis, or superficial and around the vulva. Sometimes the pain follows infection, sometimes it is as a result of vaginismus, and sometimes it results from attempts at intercourse before arousal.

Gynaecologists usually examine carefully to rule out tiny abnormalities. This may include a small operation under a general anaesthetic when the surgeon looks inside the abdomen to make sure that there are no problems deep inside the pelvis.

Sexual phobias
Most people have some form of phobia. A common one is of spiders, but phobias can develop over sexual problems, with women being unable to tolerate the thought of touching their partner, or their partner touching them, or semen going inside them or over them.

Sexual problems in men
Sexual problems in men are broadly similar to those of women, although perhaps one important difference is that men find it hard to fake interest. An erection is either there

or it isn't, and if it is not, it is difficult to pretend that it is.

Impaired sexual interest

Everybody at some stage of their lives loses interest in sex. Men rarely admit to this; they are assumed by everyone to be always ready and willing to perform, and rarely want anyone to know they are not living up to the stereotype. Impaired sexual interest can lead to failure to get an erection, and this might be a more acceptable reason for asking for help.

Breastfeeding in women makes the level of the hormone prolactin go high in the blood, which helps milk production, but also switches off the ovary, reduces sexual desire, and makes arousal difficult. The same problem can happen in men, though without the stimulus of breastfeeding. The pituitary can secrete abnormal amounts of prolactin, either in response to some drugs such as tranquilizers or those used to treat high blood pressure, or because there is a small tumour there. Prolactin reduces sexual drive as well as fertility.

Erectile dysfunction

This is one of the commonest problems men admit to. Erection depends on many factors, and is vulnerable to drugs, alcohol, diseases of nerves and blood vessels, and psychological factors (the latter are themselves often related to education). All men at some stage of their lives have a failure of erection, and this is commoner amongst older men than younger. (This is partly because ageing leads to minor damage in the nerves and blood vessels, which impairs erection, and partly because everything else becomes more common the longer you live.) If a man with failure of erection worries unduly about it, and believes that one failure is the beginning of the end, then every time he begins to get aroused he will subconsciously inhibit his own erection.

Premature ejaculation

Rapid ejaculation is common, especially for young men having their first few attempts at vaginal intercourse; after this they develop some control and begin to be able to delay ejaculation. It has been argued that rapid ejaculation is the biological norm, and that slow intercourse with a delay in ejaculation is almost a disease of civilization. The reasoning is that Neanderthal man needed to ejaculate rapidly, because during intercourse he was vulnerable to attack from predators or enemies. Men who ejaculate rapidly are thus behaving naturally and normally. But just as Neanderthal patterns of behaviour are no longer acceptable in other activities, so most people believe that sexually we should evolve.

But when is ejaculation premature? Obviously there is a problem if ejaculation always occurs before penetration, or after the first few seconds. But Kinsey reported that three-quarters of all men ejaculated less than two minutes after entering their wives. Does that mean there should be time-limits on the different phases of sexual behaviour?

Perhaps a better definition of premature ejaculation is to suggest that it is only a problem when both partners think it is. Some couples are happy with rapid intercourse and ejaculation, either all of the time or occasionally, whilst others feel cheated if sex does not last long enough for both to get some enjoyment.

Premature ejaculation is usually present from the first sexual encounter, and is often associated with feelings of guilt. Some sex therapists believe that some men use premature ejaculation as a way of avoiding sex, on the grounds that if you make anything uninteresting you decrease desire for it.

Some couples abandon foreplay to concentrate on vaginal penetration, or try alcohol to deaden sensation, or the man tries to distract himself by thinking of things other than his partner. None of these treatments work and the first two especially often make things worse. Premature ejaculation sometimes follows stress, and sometimes is a result of sexual abstinence; the first ejaculations after a period of waiting often happen rapidly.

Retarded ejaculation
This problem is uncommon. It can follow drug treatment,

or physical disease. Ejaculation may never occur, or may occur only after prolonged stimulation, or may not occur with a partner but only with masturbation.

Some men appear not to ejaculate, even though they feel they have climaxed. This may be because they actually ejaculate into the bladder. There are some drugs and diseases that cause this, but the commonest reason is surgery to the bladder or prostate, or somewhere close by, which damages the nerves that control the muscles that close off the outlet to the bladder during ejaculation.

Ejaculatory pain or painful intercourse
This is common in women (see page 64), and rare in men. It can follow infection, either in the bladder and urinary tract or in the penis or accessory sexual organs. One expert has suggested that there is a condition in men similar to vaginismus, in that when the pelvic muscles go into spasm, usually because of worry about sex, it can lead to pain. Pain with erection or intercourse can also follow damage to, or constriction of, the foreskin. Sometimes such pain only occurs on erection, or only with penetration. Circumcision is usually the simplest treatment.

Men (or women) practising anal intercourse can have pain on entry, resulting from local infections, tears, or muscular spasm.

Erotic orchialgia is a condition which generally affects young men. If they have intense sexual arousal without orgasm the pelvic congestion that develops can result in a lot of pain which usually settles on orgasm.

Sexual phobias
These can develop in men as well as women, although they are said to be less common in men, who can become phobic about their partners touching them, or touching their partners.

Dealing with sexual problems
A few decades ago the only treatment for sexual problems was to ignore them, and hope they went away, or have

PLISSIT
• Permission
• Limited Instruction
• Specific Suggestions
• Intensive Therapy

Common sexual myths
1. A man always wants and is always ready to have sex.
2. Sex must only ever occur at the instigation of the man.
3. Any woman who initiates sex is immoral.
4. Sex equals intercourse: anything else does not really count.
5. When a man gets an erection it is bad for him not to use it to get an orgasm very soon.
6. Sex should always be natural and spontaneous: thinking or talking about it spoils it.
7. All physical contact must lead to intercourse.
8. Men should not express their feelings.
9. Any man knows how to give pleasure to any woman.
10. Sex is really good only when partners have orgasms simultaneously.
11. If people love each other they know how to enjoy sex together.
12. Partners in a sexual relationship instinctively know what the other partner thinks or wants.
13. Masturbation is dirty or harmful.

several years of personal, in-depth, expensive, and largely irrelevant, unsuccessful, pyschotherapy.

The change has come with the work that started with sex researchers in the United States, who showed that sexual problems are common, usually have a simple explanation, and can be cured with simple treatments. The treatments are largely behavioural; in other words, they alter the bad patterns of sexual behaviour that have developed. More recent treatments use modern medical and surgical techniques to deal with the problems of the menopause, the problems of failure to achieve an erection, and the problems of painful intercourse.

Counselling for sexual problems

Treatment of sexual problems has changed radically over the past two decades. Sexual counselling is successful, but one of the most important things that counsellors say is that much of their work is undoing poor education, myths, and similar problems. Education is one of the most important sides of their work.

Training you to be a counsellor is beyond the scope of this book, but in essence much work is based on the acronym PLISSIT. This stands for Permission, Limited Instruction, Specific Suggestions, and Intensive Therapy.

Most couples simply require the knowledge that they are otherwise normal, and limited teaching to overcome small areas of difficulty. Few need intensive therapy. Most people are now prepared to discuss the communication problems which once led to misery.

Education usually begins with describing the normal sexual response together with explaining that many of the myths about sexuality are just that. If there are obvious medical or psychological problems, these need to be treated by an appropriate specialist. For example, a sexual problem may be linked to the drugs mentioned earlier that interfere with erection or arousal. Some men find that cigarette smoking interferes with erection, which becomes normal when they stop smoking. If people say their problems seem to get better when they drink alcohol it suggests that they are anxious; when that anxiety is relieved things often get better. Anxiety can be relieved by drugs, but discussion is better.

Education involves removing sexual myths. The list in the outer columns is not exhaustive, but includes many of the common ones, some of which have led to much unhappiness. Many men and women feel cheated if simultaneous orgasms do not occur, and they do not realize that vaginal intercourse does not lead to orgasm for a great many women. Some men find it impossible to believe that physical contact without intercourse is possible, and rape or sexual abuse of children leads on (for them, logically) from close, physical contact. Myth 5 is probably a link with our Neanderthal ancestors.

Treatment of sexual problems
There are no particular differences between the approaches needed for treating men or women. Both sexes are seen by counsellors, who talk about the problem, and try to understand what precipitated the decision to ask for help. Most clinics see both partners, and some use two therapists, one of each sex, who work as a team.

Women with vaginismus are taught to relax, and become happy with handling their genitals. Men with premature ejaculation are taught to recognize the signs of impending ejaculation, and then stop stimulating themselves, to prolong the plateau phase between arousal and ejaculation.

Physical treatments
Not every sexual problem responds to counselling. There are some physical problems that respond to other treatments.

The menopause
The menopause is the last of the 400 or so periods a woman has. It marks the ending of hormone production from the ovary. The lack of hormones, especially oestrogen, leads to the vulva and vagina shrinking, and many other symptoms, all of which have now yielded to oestrogen hormone replacement therapy. Giving oestrogens to women who

14. Masturbation within a sexual relationship is wrong.
15. If a man loses his erection it means he does not find his partner attractive.
16. It is wrong to have fantasies during intercourse.
17. A man cannot say 'no' to sex/a woman cannot say 'no' to sex.
18. There are certain, absolute, universal rules about what is normal in sex.
From Sex Therapy. A Practical Guide *by Keith Hawton. Published by Oxford Medical Publications.*

no longer get them from their ovaries means that their skin, breasts and bones no longer age (all of which are important for attractiveness), their vulva and vagina do not shrink and become thin, and the reflexes that give lubrication in response to arousal return to functioning normally.

Oestrogens can be given in many different forms, and women who feel they need them should either visit their doctor or a specialist menopause clinic.

Vaginal surgery

A small minority of women with either vaginismus or severe pain on intercourse have diseases of the vulva or vagina. Many decades ago a standard treatment for both conditions was an operation to make the vaginal inlet larger. Nobody believes in this approach nowadays, but where there are small areas of problems, for example warts, or scarring from infection, then removing these can help.

One uncommon condition is that of a rigid hymen. This can prevent intercourse, and in extreme cases even menstruation, and once removed with a simple surgical operation, normal sexual activity can occur.

Penile prostheses

Some men cannot have an erection because of permanent damage to their erectile tissue or the mechanisms that control it. There are now surgical treatments that help them. These are new, and specialized.

There are several different forms. The earliest ones used a silver bar surgically implanted in the penis and running down the length of it. The man concerned had a permanent erection, which he could conceal by bending his penis upwards and strapping it to his abdomen. Later treatments used a silastic (silicone plastic) splint, and the most modern versions are now hollow, made of silicone, and can be pumped up. This means that most of the time the man does not have an erection, but when he wants one he uses the pump to give himself one. And believe it or not, most people cannot tell the difference between one of these erections and a 'natural' one.

All of these devices are expensive, all seem to be successful, but all of them damage the erectile tissue of the penis. This means that once they have been fitted they need to be left in for life, because removing them is not possible without destroying the capacity of the penis for erection (unless of course another splint is used).

Penile injections

Erection of the penis follows changes in the blood flow through erectile tissue. These changes can be produced easily, by injecting drugs into the shaft of the penis. This is a simple procedure, done by the man in the privacy of his home, using the same sort of syringe that diabetics use to inject themselves with insulin. The injection is virtually painless, and will produce a firm erection that lasts for several hours before gradually resolving.

Unavoidable conditions

This book has described some of the ways you can keep your sex life healthy, and prevent the problems that can spoil your happiness. But not every condition that affects sex is preventable. What then? What do you do if something over which you have no control strikes you? The rest of this book will discuss such problems.

There is a temptation to include ageing in this section. Whilst ageing, and the physical effects it produces, is unavoidable, there is no reason for this to affect the sexual side of your life. True, in the survey mentioned earlier, Kinsey suggested that 27% of men at the age of 70 were unable to get erections, but this still leaves the majority able to function normally sexually.

There are a few obvious changes. In men the refractory period after orgasm lasts for longer, and so it may mean that intercourse every day is no longer possible, and the plateau phase is shortened, so that ejaculation occurs more rapidly, and the volume of the ejaculate is down. Some women who have not taken additional oestrogens (and not every woman needs them, wants them, and is suited to them) may find that their genitals are tender, and less able to respond. But these are minor changes, and for many men and women sex in the mature years is better than ever before. Men and women who have always led active lives tend to preserve themselves better in the mature years.

There are some diseases that affect sexual functioning, and even more of a problem, some diseases for which the cure sometimes or always damages sensitivity. Such diseases include those where nerves or the brain degenerate. Even some of these have an avoidable element. Blood vessel disease is a common complication of high blood pressure, the Western way of life, and cigarette smoking, but by the time it is established usually little can be done, although stopping smoking, taking exercise, and watching your diet can stop it getting worse.

Other diseases may lead to loss of sexual functioning, but there are ways of helping most sufferers, and again education is important. The surgery needed for some cancers can destroy sexuality, as in the removal of the penis for cancer. Cancer of the penis is uncommon, although some scientists believe it will become more common as the virus that may cause it spreads.

Cancer can also affect sexuality indirectly. The radical operations used for treating cancer of the rectum can destroy the nerves responsible for erection. Women who lose a breast because of cancer feel less sexually attractive after the operation than before; thankfully mastectomy (the removal of a breast) is becoming less common as surgeons adopt more conservative practices. The other great advance of recent years has been the realization that silicone breasts are not the prerogative of film starlets, but the right of any woman who wants one following mutilating surgery.

Sexuality and disability

For years there was a 'them' and 'us' attitude to the disabled. Until a few decades ago, people with disability were kept hidden from view. There are dozens of stories of rich families who kept a disturbed child or parent locked away in an attic. Much more common were the grand institutions set in acres of countryside that provided asylum for those whom society wished not to see.

Society now realizes that disabled people are in most ways the same as the rest of the population. They are simply people with a disability, but they have the same needs as others.

Disabled people may get food and shelter in the residential homes, but in them they are denied sensible employment, or control over their daily lives, or any form of sexuality. This is despite the fact that they have the same urges and desires for love, affection, and sexual fulfilment as the rest of society. Those in society who are not handicapped, and are not segregated at school or work, find sexual relief relatively easy to get. Masturbation can be almost impossible if you are physically disabled, and a satisfying sexual relationship impossible if your custodians are terrified that you may want to breed, or defile their women. Even for those who overcome many of these difficulties, part of building a relationship is normal social development. Those who have been disabled and isolated from an early age are unlikely to have developed the social and emotional skills that are necessary to start a relationship, much less to consummate it.

These prejudices explain in part why many people oppose care in the community of disabled people; hidden away they are less of a threat to us, less of a reminder that any of us may one day be disabled, or have a disabled child.

Not all societies treat their disabled members in this way. In some, they are simply killed, perhaps by being abandoned as babies. Others revere them. In Ancient Rome some disabled people held special roles as soothsayers; they were believed to be under the direct influence of a particular god, who marked them out from the rest of society. Skeletons have been found from Stone Age burial mounds, indicating that these nomadic communities kept their disabled with them as they moved round the countryside, although the lack of written records means we do not know if they kept them with them as a social act or because they believed them to be godly.

Sex aids

Almost everybody in Britain will use some form of artificial aid at some stage in their life. Short-sighted people use spectacles, those who have had a leg amputated think nothing of arranging for an artificial one, and a frighteningly high number of people use dentures. But the thought of sex aids upsets many, and this is inhibiting for those who need them. It also makes them vulnerable to exploitation. The type of shoddy workmanship that would not be tolerated on an artificial limb is almost universal in vibrators: few people would dare to complain about this to their local Trading Standards Officer.

Sex aids range from the simple and obvious to the more elaborate. A woman with arthritis, or whose partner is arthritic, may put a pillow under the small of her back to make penetration easier. Men and women with physical difficulties may need assistance with masturbation, either with a vibrator or an artificial vagina. Incidentally, it is now possible for doctors working in the United Kingdom to prescribe these for their patients under the National Health Service.

The rest of this section will discuss particular diseases that may disable partially or completely, and the effect they have on sex life.

Loss of sensation

There are five senses. Smell and taste are important sexually, but losing either does not impose a great handicap, although interestingly enough, mentally handicapped girls without the sense of smell are said never to menstruate. Much more important are the senses involved in communication. Leaving aside Dorothy Parker's fatuous comment that 'Men seldom make passes/At girls who wear glasses' which is obviously not true, blind or partially-sighted people are less able to meet others, and respond less well, or not at all, to their visual signals. Similarly, deaf people have a reputation for being standoffish; it is simply that like the blind, others may find it difficult to communicate with them.

Mental handicap

Mental handicap is common, and arouses fears amongst the rest of the population. Some mentally handicapped people are sexually aggressive; but so are some of the rest of the population. Similarly, some people believe that mentally handicapped men expose themselves, or sexually interfere with children. These practices are also found in the rest of the population. Mentally handicapped people who act in this way may do so because of their handicap, but are more likely to do so because of poor, or no, education in sexual matters, their isolation, and the need they have to achieve some form of sexual outlet. Other groups of people confined to their own company for long periods of time, without much contact with the rest of society, and especially the opposite sex, (such as soldiers, sailors, and prisoners) do not have a reputation for chastity or even normal social graces. There is also a belief that mentally handicapped women are vulnerable to unwanted pregnancies, and in recognition of this in England and Wales the Sexual Offences Act makes it unlawful for a man to have intercourse with a woman suffering from mental subnormality severe enough to prevent her from leading an independent life or guarding herself against exploitation.

Not all mentally handicapped people are fertile or sexually active. Most men with Down's syndrome are infertile and not sexually active. Most mentally handicapped people can be taught about sexuality and the importance of not offending others, and will understand this, if the teaching is careful and repetitive. Incidentally, severe mental handicap means that both men and women are legally unable to consent to intercourse.

Most mental handicaps are not hereditary; most mentally handicapped children are born to parents of normal intelligence.

Cerebral palsy

Cerebral palsy is a condition where brain damage either before, during, or shortly after, birth leads to permanent damage. Sufferers were once called spastics; this term is not used now because many of them do not in fact have spasticity, but other muscle defects, which are often more isolating. The able-bodied can usually cope with the sight of someone in a wheel-chair, but find it much harder to accept someone with a body that is continually writhing, or who has repeated facial tics; it can be even more difficult if the person has a speech defect or is partially blind as well. Intellectually these people are normal, and they usually have normal sex drives and capacity for sex. There is no reason for them not to become parents, but poor control of their bodies may make intercourse difficult, and in women uncontrolled reflexes and body movements can make labour difficult.

Paraplegia

Paraplegia is the condition that follows damage to the

spinal cord. The spinal cord is protected by the vertebrae (the backbone) and not every broken back leads to paraplegia. Once it has developed, paraplegia is usually permanent.

Men and women with paraplegia are unable to have orgasms because an orgasm is the response the brain makes to signals from the genitals, and when the spinal cord is damaged there is no way the genital signals can reach the brain. Both men and women with paraplegia have normal sex drives. Men with paraplegia are often infertile, usually because the altered blood flow to the scrotum warms the testes and so affects the development of spermatozoa, which is temperature sensitive. Women with paraplegia are as fertile as they were before the accident, but usually have no periods for the first few months after the accident. When they go into labour they can develop all sorts of abnormal reflexes that can be dangerous, especially if the reflexes raise their blood pressure.

It is possible for men with paraplegia to have erections. These erections are not under the control of their brain, and so do not occur when they see an attractive person, or have sexual thoughts. They occur when the nerves around the penis are stimulated. This can be by manual masturbation, but the intense stimulation needed is usually best achieved by using a vibrator. Such vibrators should be bought from an electrical goods shop or a pharmacy, where they are sold as body massagers, because these have more power than the flimsy battery-powered vibrators available from sex shops.

Epilepsy

Epilepsy is a condition where the brain sends abnormal signals to the muscles, which twitch or convulse as a consequence. People with epilepsy are of normal intelligence, but because they need drugs for as long as they have the condition there are some effects on sexuality.

The first is that for some convulsions occur when they are excited. This is uncommon, but can obviously inhibit sexuality. Also, the drugs they need to take to prevent convulsions may reduce sex drive, and the ability to have an orgasm, as well as making ejaculation less likely to occur.

Diabetes

Diabetes is common. It is a disease where there is interference with the control of the levels of blood sugars and fats, and one consequence of it is premature ageing of blood vessels and nerves.

Many men and women with diabetes have sexual difficulties. So do many men and women who do not have diabetes, but sexual problems seem to be a little more common amongst those with diabetes, especially poorly treated diabetes.

There are several possible reasons for this. The first is physical; if the nerves or blood vessels supplying the pelvis have begun to degenerate, then it is logical to expect that they will function less well.

The second reason is less tangible. Anyone with a disease that may shorten his or her life, which also requires regular urine testing, and careful attention to diet, may find the constant reminder of mortality oppressive, making sexual desires irrelevant.

But the third reason is more worrying. Everybody, at some stage of their lives, has a sexual problem. It is usually something temporary; not getting on well with your partner, or too much alcohol, or a bad dose of influenza. But some diabetics, when they mention this, are told that it is something inevitable, to be expected, and probably means the end of their sex lives. It doesn't, but it certainly does their self-esteem no good.

Strokes

A stroke is the most feared complication of high blood pressure or blood vessel disease. It implies that one of the small blood vessels in the brain has burst, or become blocked, and that the part of the brain supplied by that blood vessel has died. This might be a relatively unimportant part of the brain, or it might be the part which gives some of the capacity for thought, or the area responsible for controlling movement. Strokes are common, and can reduce the most independent and active of us to a life in hospital or an institution, in a matter of moments.

Sexual problems become common after any major disease or admission to hospital. Men may lose the ability to have an erection, and women may be unable to lubricate, but these difficulties are usually transient.

After the initial illness convalescence begins. Those who make a full recovery will probably have no long-term problems, but much more likely is an incomplete recovery with some permanent disabilities. These may be relatively minor, such as premature ejaculation following intensi- fied reflexes in men. More of a problem is control of either the bowels or the bladder, especially in men. There are few things more upsetting than incontinence in a partner. Men with urinary problems may need to use a modified condom system or intermittent self-catheterization (plac- ing a plastic tube into the bladder up the penis). This will obviously prevent any form of sexual activity with the penis.

Arthritis

Arthritis is common, and affects people in a wide variety of ways. One diseased joint being painful can have almost no significant effect, but disease affecting almost every joint is crippling. It can mean restriction of movements of the fingers, so removing the ability for the fine play of finger movements so useful for masturbation or stimulat- ing your partner. It can also make intercourse difficult, although with experimentation most couples find at least one position which is comfortable.

Kidney failure

The kidneys are important for removing most of the poisons that the body produces, and when they fail, death occurs, unless the sufferer either receives a new kidney (kidney transplantation) or uses a kidney machine (renal dialysis), which must be used every few days for life.

Men and women with kidney failure are infertile; fertility will return for some, but not all, after transplantation. Women can become pregnant, and have normal children, after transplantation or whilst having renal dialysis. Many men are unable to have erections in either situation.

Colostomy and similar operations

Many serious diseases, not all of them cancers, are treated by these operations. A colostomy is an artificial opening of the colon on the front of the abdomen, and if it is permanent it usually implies that the anus and rectum have been removed, but this is not always the case. An ileostomy is a similar procedure, but this time the portion of the bowel brought to the skin is the ileum or small intestine. A urostomy is a procedure similar to the above, but where one or both ureters are brought to the skin. These operations are often, but not necessarily, permanent.

All of these procedures can affect sexuality. They are visible only to the partner and only when the person is undressed. It can be difficult to disentangle the psychological effects from those of the surgery needed to create the new opening, or the underlying disease that led to the surgery in the first place.

Cancer surgery

Cancer surgeons used to pride themselves on removing much normal tissue as well as cancerous tissue. They did so because they believed that this gave the best chances for survival of the patient.

Unfortunately, the damage that was, and sometimes still is, caused at the same time often made life unpleasant; careless abdominal or pelvic surgery can have a severe effect on the person's sex life. Surgeons are now becoming more selective, and as drug treatment and radiotherapy to help treat the cancer improve, so surgery is becoming more specialized. But remember that surgery also restores damaged organs, and so improves the quality of life.

To sum up

So what if disease has altered your sex life? The first thing to remember is that you are not alone, and the good thing about the changes in the attitudes of society over the past thirty years is that the medical and nursing staff, the social workers and the others involved in your care, will all be much better able to help you than they would have been in the past. They are more prepared to discuss your problems with you, and are more informed and better able to treat them. If you do have a permanent difficulty, and you cannot be helped (and there are fewer such problems these days) then remember that sex is not necessarily everything. This may be difficult to believe because of the emphasis placed on it by your friends and peers and the media. Some years ago the American agony columnist Ann Landers made this point in her column. She wrote that most women wanted more from a relationship than sex, and that if they had the choice between a man who was good at thrusting, and one who was affectionate, and caring, and close to them, and would cuddle and confide in them, they would choose the latter. She was doubted by her editors, but nearly 100,000 women wrote to her to say that she was correct.

Alternative therapies

Alternative medicine views a healthy sex life as an integral part of, and affected by, our overall health. As with other aspects of ill-health, the approach is to look at the whole person, assessing all the factors that create problems for each individual. Each therapy will therefore take into account physical, mental or emotional imbalances as well as the impact of lifestyle and the environment on health. Treatment may be in isolation, or together with other complementary or conventional approaches, and will usually include a good deal of advice on self-help measures to restore balance and prevent further problems.

Well-respected treatments of considerable value range from those dealing primarily with psychological aspects, such as hypnotherapy and psychotherapy, through energy-based therapies like acupuncture and homoeopathy, to those working more obviously on physical problems, such as herbal medicine or osteopathy. However, these may also have profound effects on mental or stress-related problems, so that this division is rather artificial and just demonstrates the variety of possible approaches.

In summary, then, alternative medical practitioners will look at each person individually, and use their particular therapy to help correct the underlying causes of imbalance which are producing sexual problems.

What can go wrong

There are many disorders that can create problems in people's sex lives. Urinary/vaginal infections such as cystitis or thrush are quite common causes of sexual dysfunction, especially for women, who more frequently suffer urinary infections. Women also often experience hormone imbalances, or functional disorders of the reproductive system such as period pains or abnormal menstrual bleeding. In men, inflammation or infection of the prostate gland or the testes, impotence or sub-fertility are some of the more obvious physical disorders which can produce difficulties.

The background reasons for these kinds of conditions are varied. For instance, there may be inadequate nutrition or malnourishment, with wide implications for the working of the immune system. Structural problems, particularly of the lower spine or the pelvic girdle, can affect the nerve and/or blood supply to the pelvic organs. Hormone imbalances may stem from the use of the contraceptive pill, or following pregnancy. Stress of one kind or another is a major factor, both in contributing to physical ill-health and directly affecting sexual desire and ability. In Chinese medicine, a fundamental imbalance in Ch'i, or vital energy, is seen as the chief underlying characteristic of such disturbances.

Thus, a variety of reasons exist for sexual problems. There are a number of viewpoints on the main predisposing factors, with a corresponding array of therapeutic approaches.

There are a number of alternative forms of treatment available. The following is a summary of the most widely-known and respected therapies. Obviously, not every treatment suits all people equally well - there are 'horses for courses' as it were. However, these therapies have a wide application for most people and many kinds of conditions.

Acupuncture
An established system of health care for several centuries, traditional Chinese medicine incorporates both acupuncture and herbalism. The basis for these therapies is the maintenance of internal harmony, or balance of energy. This harmony is usually expressed in terms of Yin/Yang, the interplay between opposing forces that can be seen in nature (e.g. heat/cold, dry/wet, hardness/softness). The flow of energy, termed Ch'i, is seen in Chinese medicine to circulate along definite pathways or channels, which form a continuous circuit linking all parts of the body. Disruption in this flow is viewed as the prime cause of ill-health.

Herbal medicine
The medicinal use of plants also extends back over

millennia, with differing systems of application being found in all cultures throughout history. Even today, it is the dominant form of treatment worldwide. Western medical herbalism combines traditional knowledge with modern clinical training and diagnostic skills, and increasingly with new research findings (many of which confirm much of the long-established actions of herbs). Like other therapies, herbal medicine is concerned with an individual, whole person approach to health, not with mere symptom relief. The aim is to assist natural healing and restore true health. Thus each person receives a unique prescription, together with appropriate advice and support.

Homoeopathy

The approach of homoeopathy, again on a unique whole-person basis, revolves around the principle of treating 'like with like'. Symptoms are seen as evidence of the person fighting the illness, and remedies are used which, if given to a healthy person, would produce symptoms that mimicked those of the patient. These remedies are, however, given in a highly diluted form called potencies. This extreme dilution makes homoeopathic medicines very safe in terms of toxicity, but they can provoke an initial aggravation of symptoms as part of the healing process. Remedies are made from a variety of sources, such as plants, minerals or animal substances. This is in contrast to herbal medicine, which only uses plant extracts from essentially non-toxic herbs, in material doses, despite occasional confusion about these two therapies.

Hypnotherapy

This is a form of treatment which can be very useful where there is a long-standing or deep-seated psychological problem underlying any condition. The aim is to induce a state of relaxation, somewhat akin to that sensation when one is half-awake in bed in the morning - perfectly conscious, but more receptive to contemplating past traumas locked away in the sub-conscious or to new, positive ideas. Many hypnotherapists are also psychotherapists and use various counselling skills as part of their work.

Naturopathy

Naturopathy is based on the principle of 'you are what you eat', at least to a great extent. Since dietary imbalances or deficiencies are important factors in both physical and emotional disorders, clinical nutrition is a valuable form of treatment. The emphasis is on changes in the diet as far as possible, with specific supplements as necessary. Dietary therapy exists in its own right, as well as being part of the approach of other therapies. In addition to diet, naturopaths may look at hydrotherapy (the use of water applications such as compresses or sitz baths) to improve circulation and elimination.

Osteopathy and chiropractic

Although these two therapies have some differences, both in diagnosis and treatment, they are both concerned in the main with manipulation of the spine and joints. Chiropractors are much more likely to take X-rays to help diagnosis, and the methods of correcting structural problems are not the same. Despite the fact that they are often thought of as 'back-care therapies', these treatments can have wider effects on health. A particularly useful time to think of them with regard to sexual problems is if there is discomfort following pregnancy and childbirth, when there may have been a tilting of the pelvis or lower spine.

In addition to the above therapies, other useful alternatives include remedial massage to relax and ease tension and improve circulation, and healing, in which the therapist acts as a 'channel' for healing energy to flow and stimulate the person's own self-correcting mechanisms.

Cystitis

This is inflammation of the bladder and is probably the commonest urinary problem. It may or may not be related to an actual infection, but the symptoms of increased frequency of urination and associated discomfort will be similar in both cases. Recurrent bouts of cystitis are quite frequent, especially among women, and lead to a chronic irritation of the lining of the bladder and also often to discomfort from intercourse.

Naturopathy

Alternative treatments are often of tremendous value, especially in recurrent cystitis. One area is nutrition, and here naturopaths and medical herbalists offer particular expertise. Advice will include looking at the intake of foods and liquids which are least irritating to the bladder tissues - avoiding or reducing alcohol, for instance - and which provide essential nutrients for local healing, such as silica. A common suggestion is the increased consumption of alkali-forming foods to raise the pH (that is, make less acidic) of the urine, especially in the acute phases of cystitis. In addition, improved nutrition for the whole body, including the immune system, circulation and nervous system, is a basic target of such therapies.

Herbalism

Herbal medicine itself can be very helpful in a variety of ways: in the acute phase urinary antiseptic and anti-inflammatory remedies will help to disinfect the urinary passages, reduce discomfort and repair the damaged tissues. For example, drinking herb teas like Chamomile eases the inflamed bladder, reduces spasm and calms the irritated tissues. Following on such treatment, herbal diuretics increase output of urine from the kidneys and speed up the removal of irritating toxins. Finally, general treatment can help to boost immunity and non-specific resistance to disease, and improve underlying health and vitality.

Homoeopathy

This general approach, looking at constitutional weaknesses, would be the main feature of homoeopathic treatment, using highly diluted remedies to stimulate the person's own healing energies in acute or chronic attacks.

Acupuncture

In quite a different way, the aim of acupuncture would be the correction of energy blockages in the short term and the balancing of the person's pattern and use of energy internally in the long term.

Osteopathy and chiropractic

The integrity of the pelvic structure and/or the lower back may be important, since accident, injury or other disorders of this area can affect the nerves and blood vessels which supply the pelvic organs. These nerves emerge from the lower lumbar and sacral vertebrae (the lower part of the spine, around the area where it meets the pelvis at the sacro-iliac joint). In addition, any structural problem here may produce direct pressure on the bladder. The manipulative therapies are of major benefit in these types of situations.

Urethritis

Apart from the bladder itself, there may be inflammation of the urethra (the tube linking the bladder with the outside of the body), which can produce similar symptoms and treatment for which would follow a similar path. Useful self-help measures include emptying the bladder after intercourse, avoiding getting chilled and perhaps taking a hot bath or using a hot-water bottle.

Further complications could include infections of the

kidneys or the vagina, or even sexually transmitted diseases. These would all affect treatment, and only registered medical practitioners can legally treat the last category.

Thrush

This is a fungal infection by the yeast Candida albicans and related strains which has become an increasingly common source of vaginal disease over the last few years. Thrush is often experienced in recurrent bouts together with cystitis. This is not only due to the shared blood or nerve supply, but the close proximity of the vaginal and urethral openings. Quite frequently, the use of antibiotics for treating bladder infections leaves the vaginal area more susceptible to fungal infection.

Other factors which can lead to repeated thrush infection include the contraceptive pill, which can affect vaginal secretions and pH (acidity/alkalinity), local deodorants which may irritate the very delicate membranes, inadequate nutrition and chronic stress. Thus advice on self-help may look at much more than local measures. There are of course many of these that can help, such as washing the vaginal area with salt water, avoiding wearing tight clothing like jeans or tights which create a warm, moist environment ideal for fungal growth, and so on.

Alternative medicine focuses not only on the local problem but also on these causative factors and the wider issues of depressed immunity.

Naturopathy and herbalism

Sound naturopathic principles of adequate nutrition and elimination at the cellular level are basic to most treatments. A therapy of significant value is herbal medicine; internal treatment, geared to individual circumstances, would be backed up by dietary or other advice and local applications. These may have anti-fungal, anti-inflammatory and/or anti-pruritic (relieving the intense itching) properties.

Homoeopathy and acupuncture

These other therapies will tend to concentrate on improving general health and vitality. With stress in particular often playing an important role in increasing susceptibility to thrush, all these approaches can be very helpful.

Vaginismus

This is a completely different kind of problem caused by spasm of the lower vaginal muscles. This may be related to infection or inflammation of the vagina, making intercourse painful, but is more usually a problem of anxiety or high levels of tension. As such, although the above therapies can help a good deal, they need to look at the psychological side even more closely than usual and counselling is an essential part of any approach.

Hypnotherapy

This is one of the alternative options to more usual forms of sex counselling which could be valuable, especially when there are deep-seated anxieties to be resolved.

Circulation problems

The basin-like shape of the pelvis, and the reduced amounts of exercise that most of us now take, mean that pelvic congestion of the circulation occurs relatively commonly nowadays. This is especially true in women and this can be a major factor in menstrual problems. Typically, there may well be excessively heavy bleeding and discomfort during a period with pain in the lower abdomen or back, or aching down into the thighs.

Exercise

Of vital importance, therefore, is exercise, and many

alternative practitioners will give advice on appropriate forms of movement - for example, it can be very beneficial to do exercises that involve inverting the pelvis. This may be achieved through performing some yoga postures, or perhaps by 'bicycling' in the air when raised on your shoulders.

Naturopathy and massage
Therapies such as naturopathy also try to increase the circulation through the area by using hot or cold compresses over the lower abdomen, to relieve congestion and stimulate blood flow. Remedial massage can also be very helpful, reducing muscle tension or spasm and encouraging blood flow through the tissues.

Osteopathy and chiropractic
The circulatory congestion may be aggravated by mechanical problems of the pelvic structure, such as tilting of the pelvis or injuries to the lumbar-sacral spine. Manipulative treatments by an osteopath or chiropractor will be specifically helpful.

Posture
This is another aspect to consider. Our sedentary lifestyles and general lack of mobility encourage congestion and engorgement

of the blood vessels of the pelvic basin, with the kind of discomfort described. A very useful form of treatment here is the Alexander technique, where each person is taught how to be aware of inefficient use of the body and how to re-educate it to move, sit etc. more effectively and without strain.

In general, then, the effective flow of blood through this area is an important factor in ensuring that all the tissues and organs are supplied with nutrients and that waste products are removed. This in turn means that the reproductive organs work as well as possible. Alternative methods of treatment can help in this respect a great deal.

Hormone disorders

Hormone imbalances can affect sexual functioning or enjoyment in many different ways; for instance, women may experience problems such as menorrhagia (excessive menstrual bleeding) or metrorrhagia (bleeding at times other than during the period), premenstrual tension and irritability, menopausal symptoms like increased dryness of the vagina, and general changes in mood. For both sexes, hormone disorder can produce infertility.

Inadequate production of stress hormones by the adrenal glands will lead to tiredness, irritability or depression, and a lack of sexual desire. Alternative medicine looks at what underlying factors are present which are disturbing the balance, rather than simply using hormone replacement. Thus, excessive or abnormal menstrual bleeding can occur for many reasons, such as pelvic circulatory congestion or anaemia or pelvic inflammation or the effects of the contraceptive pill or other drug treatment. Starting, however, with poor hormone control as a cause, then natural remedies have a valuable role. Many plants contain substances with hormone-like actions which can work directly to normalize our hormone production.

Excessive bleeding
The excessive bleeding itself can also be controlled by homoeopathic or herbal medicines or by acupuncture, each of which will in its own way strive to alter the basic causes of the problem. A likely factor is incorrect nutrition, and naturopathic principles, of adequate nourishment for each cell and the effective elimination of waste matter from it, will be of essential importance. For instance iron-deficiency

anaemia, with associated tiredness and lethargy, could be a problem and can be helped through dietary therapy.

Premenstrual syndrome

This can give rise to a whole range of symptoms, with emotional disturbances and fluid retention the main ones. One of the major reasons for the premenstrual syndrome (or PMS for short) is too rapid a fall in the levels of progesterone in comparison to those of oestrogen (the two female sex hormones). This fall is due to the corpus luteum (the body within the ovary which chiefly secretes progesterone) prematurely ceasing to function. A specific treatment for this problem involves the use of the plant Vitex agnus-castus, which increases the body's production of luteinizing hormone: this in turn directly affects the corpus luteum activity.

However, many alternative therapies can indirectly help to redress the hormone imbalance and improve the symptoms of PMS. Once again, diet is often vital, and of notable importance is the vitamin B complex especially vitamin B_6 (although this is best used in conjunction with the rest of the complex). Also

of value is magnesium, especially where depression before a period is a major symptom.

Diuretic effects, increasing the output of urine and so reducing the pressure from fluid retention, can be achieved by a number of methods - many plants, for instance, are quite potent in this respect. A reduction in the tension levels and degree of stress is another area where alternative treatments can play a large part.

The menopause

During the menopause, physical and psychological changes occur which can dramatically affect sex life. Complementary medicine pays attention to all the health effects of the hormone fluctuations at this time. The decreasing levels of oestrogen in particular can lead not only to dryness and irritation of the vagina but also to rapid falls in body calcium and magnesium levels. Nutrition is helpful, but equally as important is to maintain exercise in order to slow down the calcium loss. Relaxation-based approaches to exercise and movement, such as yoga, can also substantially improve mental attitude. Major therapies like herbal medicine, homoeopathy or acupuncture can help to cushion the effects of declining hormone levels

and assist the woman to go through the internal changes necessary to adapt to these reduced levels.

Infertility

This is another problem which can stem from a number of causes other than simply hormone imbalance, e.g. chronic pelvic inflammation. In the area of hormone control, much benefit can be gained. Both Western and Chinese herbal medicine contain a number of remedies to influence hormonal secretion, and with hormone production affected by other health factors, different therapies may be of value.

Exhaustion of the adrenal glands, with a lowering of the production of stress hormones, leads to feelings of general lethargy and irritability. This exhaustion can arise from chronic stress, both physical and mental, and these causes need to be sorted out in order to turn off the 'tap' which is draining the adrenal cortex response of hormone secretion.

A number of herbal remedies have been demonstrated to act as adaptogens, that is they improve the body's ability to maintain a response to stress without becoming tired and exhausted. The most well-known of these is ginseng, which in the short term can considerably improve stress resistance, stamina and overall energy. This gives it its reputation for increasing sexual performance, which can certainly happen, but for the reasons and causes outlined above.

Prostate disorders

Essentially there are three kinds of problem that can affect the prostate gland; inflammation of the gland (prostatitis), enlargement of the prostate gland, and cancer of the prostate gland.

Prostatitis

This occurs usually as the result of urinary infection or a sexually transmitted disease. Although the latter is not legally treatable by alternative methods, therapies such as herbal medicine, homoeopathy and acupuncture can have very beneficial results on urinary infection-produced prostate inflammation.

Prostatic enlargement

Benign (i.e. non-cancerous) enlargement of the prostate is something which affects the great majority of men as they get older, and is often seen as an inevitable part of ageing. Symptoms include dribbling or reduced flow of urine,

getting up in the night and a lessening of sexual performance, especially erection. Quite frequently, the background reason is too quick a drop in the levels of testosterone (the male hormone) and this can be prevented by continuing to remain physically, and indeed sexually, active as long as possible. Again, the above therapies can be of considerable value.

Prostatic cancer

This represents only a tiny percentage of prostate enlargement causes, and is often distinguished by the speed of onset of symptoms, possibly with blood in the urine and increasing lower back or pelvic pain. Any complementary treatments are likely to be in conjunction with conventional treatment, and as with any tumour it is difficult to assess the outcome, but it is worth stating that there are possibilities for help.

Stress

Stress can affect people's sex lives in a number of ways. Long periods of being over-tired and exhausted very easily, lead to a lessening of sexual desire, or ability to be aroused. Anxiety can also make love-making itself more difficult - performance anxiety

may affect men or women, making erection difficult or ejaculation premature, or make intercourse painful. Tension and irritability can spill over into a relationship with effects on desire for and enjoyment of sex.

The first thing to say about stress is that prevention is much better than cure. Looking carefully at the ways in which we create our own stress situations, and seeking to alter some of these patterns is of prime importance. Often it needs someone else to clarify them and give guidance on how to change, and many therapies will deal with this aspect. In addition, finding suitable methods of dealing with excessive amounts of stress as well as releasing tension is very much part of the overall approach of alternative medicine.

Relaxation, yoga and massage

Most of us create stress by trying to do things at too speedy a pace, and relaxation is a key principle. This can be achieved in different ways - exercises such as yoga are particularly good at reducing physical tension and inducing a calmer attitude. Massage is another excellent way to unravel knots of tension and unwind, posture and breathing techniques can be very helpful, and so on. One of the chief tenets of alternative medicine is the re-education of people concerning lifestyle in general and our own responsibility for much of our health, so most of the therapies discussed will give appropriate advice or refer to others for more specific help.

Other disciplines

Coping better with high levels of stress is another area where other therapies can be valuable. The range of adaptogenic plant remedies has already been mentioned, and these represent a real alternative to treatments with conventional drugs etc. The use of hypnotherapy in this field is also well-recognized, and equally valuable can be acupuncture or homoeopathy. In some cases, an ability to withstand stresses may be affected by structural lesions causing pressure on the brain or spinal column, and the manipulative therapies will be called for. A form of osteopathic treatment called cranial osteopathy is of particular use where skeletal imbalance causes a blockage in our flow of internal energy and natural bio-rhythms.

Generally, then, alternative treatments have a lot to offer for stress-related sexual problems, both in terms of giving information and advice, and in providing treatment to help the individual cope and

Impotence

Impotence, or the inability of the male to maintain an erection and have sex, is largely a psychological problem, i.e. it is usually a matter of the emotional and mental attitude towards lovemaking, in particular 'performance anxiety', which is the root of the problem and not any direct physical disability.

In the majority of instances, information is needed about the nature of the problem plus reassurances that nothing is intrinsically wrong with the reproductive organs. This is an approach that is common to all the therapies and relies more on the skill and understanding of the individual practitioner than any form of treatment or medication.

There are instances, however, when psychological problems go somewhat deeper, perhaps from some trauma earlier in life, and different approaches may be of use. For instance, hypnotherapy can be appropriate - getting into the right kind of relaxed state to 'replay' a traumatic experience or work through an unresolved problem. Acupuncture can also be effective in releasing these locked-in blockages, and if difficulties have come about

from an accident say, then manipulation can have a profound effect in releasing the shock from the tissues and helping people to rebalance themselves.

Nearly every culture has had its plant-based approach to impotence and loss of sexual drive, but the aphrodisiac reputation of such remedies, in the narrow sense of the word, is often misleading. However, there are a range of herbs which can have significant effects on hormone production and on general vitality.

This latter quality is really the key to an improved sex life anyway, so that changes can be profound over time. The effects of such remedies as ginseng on stress hormone levels, stamina and overall energy, as already discussed, are the foundation for their deserved reputation in this field. The Chinese have been keen on the sex-drive stimulating aspects of herbal medicines for centuries and much of the modern research has been conducted there - and there are a lot of Chinese people! Equally, there are plants which appear to be of value in reducing excessive sex drive in men, e.g. hops, which are both a relaxant to the central nervous system and contain oestrogenic principles which curb excess testosterone production.

The effects of age

As we get older, various physical and mental changes take place which can affect our vigour and sex lives. Ageing is not in itself a problem medically, and many people continue to have active sex lives well into retirement. Although growing older is not preventable, some of the problems that are often associated with it can be lessened or prevented to a great extent.

Deterioration of the nervous system is a slow, steady consequence of age, but damage to the nerve supply can occur through incorrect nutrition, the intake of alcohol or tobacco, or from long-term drug use. Similarly, the state of our blood vessels can be significantly aggravated by smoking in particular, and liver function can be disturbed by alcohol or drug intake. All these physical changes can be ameliorated by changes in habit as well as therapeutic help.

Nutrition

In terms of diet, an adequate supply of vitamins, minerals and trace elements is essential to ensure proper functioning of the mind and body. As examples, vitamin B is vital for nerve activity and vitamin E has valuable effects on maintaining the elasticity of the skin and blood vessel walls; garlic has a well-documented use in lowering blood cholesterol levels, as well as boosting the immune system and energy. Vitamin C, destroyed by smoking, is also vital for resistance to disease and stress, and is needed on a daily basis.

Herbal treatments

Herbal medicines are useful in a number of wide-ranging ways from regenerating liver cells damaged by drug, alcohol or other poisoning to improving circulation and digestion (most traditional tonics were based on the use of bitters to stimulate digestive and liver function) to nervine and adaptogenic remedies for overall effects on mental and physical vigour.

Homoeopathy and acupuncture

These disciplines each address the constitution of the individual, stimulating the person's own energies and self-correcting abilities. Encouraging someone to continue with an active physical and mental lifestyle is a central piece of advice for most therapies, and regular sexual activity is certainly useful in prolonging one's sex life.

Some of the specific problems that may occur with ageing, such as dryness of the vagina, have been covered under Hormone Disorders and are not in themselves insuperable without hormone replacement. Differing attitudes to sexual activity as one gets older, and the emphasis on the wider benefits of the relationship can make sex life very rewarding at any age.

Infertility

Infertility is not one problem, but several. In men, there may be a low sperm count or production of non-viable sperm, while for women the problems may be low or abnormal egg production, an internal environment which is hostile to the sperm, or the fertilized egg may not be able to be retained. Infertility is only permanent in a minority of people who have been diagnosed as infertile with frequent instances of 'spontaneous recovery' i.e. the woman becomes pregnant.

One of the chief causes of infertility is an imbalance in the endocrine system, and the contribution that alternative medicine can play in correcting hormone disorders has been discussed on page 89. Dysfunction of the ovaries or testes can certainly respond in many circumstances to these therapies.

Also of frequent importance is chronic pelvic inflammation,

a low-grade infection or inflammation of the pelvic organs especially in women. The inflammation can be set up by a number of local problems, such as any kind of infection or perhaps a sexually transmitted disease, scar tissue following childbirth or operation, abortion or indeed simply the use of the coil for contraception. The symptoms include unusually bad pain with periods, ovulation and intercourse, a discharge and/or menorrhagia (heavy bleeding). The risk of the fallopian tubes getting blocked and causing infertility increases with time and degree of the inflammation.

However, all this should not be seen as too negative; treatments to improve non-specific resistance to disease and the functioning of the ovaries can, over time, effect a considerable change in the problem - from the plant world for instance, the herb Chamaelirium luteum appears to have an adaptogenic effect on the ovaries, regulating their actions. Each of the major forms of alternative medicine has its own methods and potential for helping to correct the problem, and without giving false hope to would-be parents who appear to be infertile there is a good deal of scope for assistance among the complementary disciplines.

Relationship difficulties

For many people, their sexual relationships are severely affected by wider aspects of their inability to relate to one another, their self-image or changes in their lifestyle. Of the latter, probably the most common is pregnancy and childbirth; the woman finds her body has altered dramatically to fulfil the needs of nurturing the fetus and then breastfeeding the baby, with a shift in the relationship to include being a mother as well. Similarly, the man has to adapt to these changes in her body and use of the breasts, all in the context of being part of a larger family group.

Whether for this reason, or because of other difficulties in developing physical relationships, many people find that they need to relearn how to share touching and sexual enjoyment. The most obvious form of help in this context is sexual counselling, which may well need solely to be information and reassurance that there is not an intractable problem and advice on ways to change. There is quite a bit of scope for other complementary approaches to assist as well.

Massage
One of the therapies with particular benefit is massage, both therapeutically to aid relaxation as well as getting people back in tune with their bodies. It is also taught for use at home as part of re-establishing physical contact.

Self-image
On a more general note, the question of self-image can bring in all kinds of health problems, e.g. skin diseases, and herbal, homoeopathic or acupuncture treatments are viable alternatives for many of these conditions. Problems with physical relations are often bound up with reactions to one's own appearance or health, and these can be as significant as the disorder itself.

Quite obviously, the mental and emotional side can be tackled by several approaches, such as hypnotherapy or psychotherapy or the different styles of healing. Therefore, the need to look at the whole person is paramount, since basic physical imbalances can be a part of the emotional problem, and a combination of approaches may be most appropriate.

Sexually transmitted diseases
In Britain, it is illegal for anyone other than a registered medical practitioner to treat sexually transmitted diseases.

In times past, of course, there were a number of herbal remedies that were used to treat such problems, and homoeopathy and acupuncture have historically been used also. There is certainly scope for complementary treatments to help alleviate symptoms associated with these diseases, while the problem itself is treated conventionally.

A general principle is the boosting of overall immunity, strengthening the body's defences against further infection, and also discouraging spread of the condition - again, any known contacts should also seek medical advice or treatment from a doctor or special clinic. The three therapies mentioned above present probably the most likely alternative ways to encourage such immune stimulation, with some plants, such as Echinacea angustifolia, demonstrating very positive results in this field.

Some sexually transmitted diseases can give rise to secondary problems, such as urinary infections or pelvic inflammation, and these may well be treatable by alternative means (see the relevant sections for further details). Attention to nutrition and hygiene are basic standard self-help measures that are likely to be suggested alongside any treatment - salt baths or washes for the genital area can be very useful in this respect.

AIDS

Of particular significance in recent years has been the development of AIDS, and this is a problem where alternative therapies can be of significant value in many ways. Although AIDS is associated with infection by the Human Immunodeficiency Virus (HIV), this is only a part of the overall picture, and alternative medicine pays attention to a wide range of stresses on our immune systems, such as drugs, alcohol, diet, stress, the environment etc.

Most of the information concerning the uses and value of other treatments for AIDS and the AIDS Related Complex (ARC) comes from the United States, and there the main therapies which have been shown to be of benefit in containing ARC symptoms have been herbal medicine, especially Chinese herbs, and acupuncture. A major difficulty with any treatment has been the rather erratic way in which the sufferers tend to adhere to any form of therapy, and their tendency to use several approaches at once; there is some scope, however, for real hope of a positive immuno-tonic benefit from these treatments.

Lack of energy

A combination of excessive tiredness, lethargy and a general lack of energy is one of the commonest reasons for decreasing interest in sex in a relationship and for lowering sex drive generally. Tiredness is in itself a symptom, and there are many factors which can be responsible, from chronic stress (also see Stress section) to a number of ailments or imbalances.

Nutritional medicine

On a nutritional level, there can be several deficiencies - iron-deficiency anaemia is an obvious example - which can be corrected by dietary change or supplementation. Many substances, such as brewer's yeast, Royal Jelly, Ginseng etc. have been promoted over the years for their energy-giving properties and this is in part due to their replacement of a simple lack of vitamins, minerals or trace elements. A slightly different problem, which can be related to a nutritional lack, and improved by extra dietary iodine, especially the use of kelp, is an imbalance of the thyroid gland.

Another condition which gives rise to great tiredness is hypoglycaemia, or low blood sugar levels, and this is in varying degrees really quite common. Again, great benefit can be achieved by dietary change; usually, there is a pattern of eating foods rich in sugar but low in fibre, which places considerable stress on the liver and pancreas to try and stabilize blood sugar levels.

Myalgic encephalomyelitis

One of the most significant health problems to have been recognized in recent years is M.E. (myalgic encephalomyelitis, often called post-viral fatigue syndrome). The predominant symptom of this distressing condition is the intense fatigue and total lack of energy, often for several years. This is a problem where alternative medicine has a lot to offer.

Herbal medicines

As far as herbal medicine goes, differing approaches may be necessary for the above and other debilitating conditions. The use of stimulating remedies is likely to be short-term, if at all, and tonic or nervous restorative remedies are much more frequently of benefit. Liver tonics, bitters and the like could be called for to improve the digestion and regulate blood sugar or energy levels. Improvements to the circulation will often be helpful - as always, each person is

treated individually.

Acupuncture and homoeopathy

Acupuncture, and in a different way homoeopathy, are directly concerned with the flow and use of energy by the body, and can address the problem by re-establishing a correct pattern of energy distribution. Other disciplines, such as massage, shiatsu (occasionally called acupressure) and reflexology may also be of assistance in rebalancing our bodies.

Osteopathy and chiropractic

Naturally, if there is any structural imbalance which is causing fatigue, for instance as a result of constant pain or stiffness of movement, then osteopathy or chiropractic may well be the most appropriate treatments to consider.

Psychotherapy and hypnotherapy

Tiredness can come about because of a general dissatisfaction with life, perhaps a boring, undemanding job or depression over some problem, and the main therapies initially discussed above can be helpful in lifting the mood: there can also be scope for help by counselling, perhaps using psychotherapy or hypnotherapy, to work on

the mental and emotional side of things in a more concentrated way.

Other disorders that could contribute to a lack of energy and thus a lowered sex drive, usually developing later on in life, include hypertension (high blood pressure), adult onset diabetes, obesity and gall stones. As always it is through the investigation of the individual circumstances that alternative therapies will determine whether and how they can help. From insomnia to immune-system depression, a sense of fatigue has a variety of causes and demonstrates that sex life and general health are inextricably bound up together, each contributing to the other for a more fulfilling life.

Other titles in the series

Your Pregnancy and Childbirth
(ISBN 0 245-55068-2)
Your Active Body (ISBN 0 245-55070-4)
Your Heart and Lungs (ISBN 0 245-55069-0)

Available, Spring 1990
Your Mind (ISBN 0 245-60008-6)
Your Diet (ISBN 0 245-60009-4)
Your Skin (ISBN 0 245-60010-8)
Your Child (ISBN 0 245-60011-6)

Available, Autumn 1990
Your Female Body (ISBN 0 245-60012-4)
Your Senses (ISBN 0 245-60013-2)
A-Z of Conditions and Drugs (ISBN 0 245-60014-0)

Further reading

Some of these books are referred to in the text. They expand on the subjects already touched upon.

Contraception. The Facts. Peter Bromwich and Tony Parsons. Published by Oxford University Press 1984; republished 1989.

Family Doctor Guides. Menopause. Peter Bromwich. Published by Equation and the British Medical Association 1989.

Progress in Obstetrics and Gynaecology. Edited by John Studd. Volume 7, 1989. Chapter 14. The sex ratio and ways of manipulating it. Published by Churchill Livingstone.

Sex Therapy. A practical guide. Keith Hawton. Published by Oxford Medical Publications 1985.

Private Parts. A health book for men. Yosh Taguchi. Published by Macdonald Optima 1988.

The Male Member. Kit Schwartz. Published by Robson Books 1988.

Useful organizations

*Family Planning Association Information Service
27-35 Mortimer Street
London W1N 7RJ*

*Women's Health and Reproductive Rights Information Centre
52-54 Featherstone Street
London EC1Y 8RT*

*British Chiropractic Association
Premier House
10 Greycoat Place
London SW1P 1SB*

*Council for Acupuncture (umbrella group for the main colleges)
Suite One
191A Cavendish Square
London W1M 9AD*

*General Council and Register of Osteopaths
56 London Street
Reading
Berkshire RG21 4SQ*

*National Institute of Medical Herbalists
41 Hatherley Road
Winchester
Hampshire SO22 6RR*

*PRIME HEALTH
Prime House
Barnett Wood Lane
Leatherhead
Surrey KT22 7BS
0372 386060*